DYSPRAXIA AND ITS MANAGEMENT

Dyspraxia and its Management

N. Miller

Speech Therapist
Belfast Hospital for Sick Children
Belfast
Ireland (North)

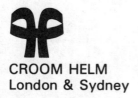

CROOM HELM
London & Sydney

Croom Helm Ltd, Provident House, Burrell Row,
Beckenham, Kent BR3 1AT
Croom Helm Auatralia Pty Ltd, Suite 4, 6th Floor,
64-76 Kippax Street, Surry Hills, NSW 2010, Australia

British Library Cataloguing in Publication Data

Miller, Niklas
    Dyspraxia and its management.
    1. Movement disorders
    I. Title
    616.7   RC925
    ISBN 0-7099-3553-6

Filmset by Mayhew Typesetting, Bristol, England
Printed and bound in Great Britain
by Billing & Sons Limited, Worcester.

CONTENTS

Acknowledgements

1. Introduction   1

2. The Gestural Dyspraxias   16
   Ideational Dyspraxia   17
   Ideomotor Dyspraxia   25
   Modality Specific Dyspraxia   36
   Sympathetic Dyspraxia   37
   Differential Diagnosis   40
   Oral-facial Dyspraxia   46

3. Constructional Dyspraxia   56

4. Apraxia of Speech   90

5. Ocular-motor Apraxia   115
   Congenital   115
   Acquired   125

6. Dyspraxia-related Disturbances   128
   Callosal Dyspraxia   128
   Frontal Dyspraxia   136
   Axial Movements and Dyspraxia   140
   Gait Dyspraxia   143
   Dressing Dyspraxia   149

7. Developmental Dyspraxia   155

8. Therapy   195

Glossary   217

Bibliography   220

Author Index   235

Subject Index   241

for R.C.I.M.J.B.

to my father on his seventieth birthday

ACKNOWLEDGEMENTS

While accepting responsibility for shortcomings of the final version of this book, thanks have to go to many friends and colleagues from the nursing, paramedical and medical fields who gave valuable support and suggestions to help the work to completion. They are, unfortunately, too numerous to mention individually. I am grateful to Mr T. Buchanan for discussion about the ocular-motor dyspraxia chapter, and to Miss M. Edwards, who commented on earlier versions of the oral and speech dyspraxia chapters. Dr S. Hawkins and Vera Blair commented on drafts of the gestural dyspraxias sections. R. Sage offered advice on developmental dyspraxia. Brendan Ellis produced the fine drawings from the video recordings.

There were several colleagues who gave especial assistance: Mildred Saunders and her staff in the Clinical Library of the Victoria Hospital, Belfast, dealt kindly, patiently and efficiently with my constant demands to track down books and articles from the most distant and obscure sources; Marlene Law put up sympathetically and constructively with the endless questions and preliminary versions of chapters inflicted on her; my speech therapy colleague Margaret Newman not only gave helpful hints on various parts of the book, but enabled the work to be completed within the allotted time and tolerance span by generously taking over some of my clinical responsibilities.

Most of all, thanks are due to my family near and far for the love and support they have given throughout the writing of the book. To my mother even greater thanks are due for the mammoth task of typing and retyping the entire manuscript. Those who have not undertaken such a project probably feel that authors always name their family under acknowledgement just to give them a free mention. Those who have undertaken such works will realise that the full thanks can never be expressed in mere words.

N. Miller
Béal Feirste
Bealtaine

1 INTRODUCTION

As for the flight of a bullet, or a shell or bomb fragment, that rips open a man's skull, splitting and burning the tissues of his brain, crippling his memory, sight, hearing, awareness — these days people don't find anything extraordinary in that. But if it's not extraordinary, why am I ill? . . . It's depressing having to start all over and make sense out of a world you've lost because of injury and illness, to get these bits and pieces to add up to a coherent whole.

L. Zasetsky (Luria, 1982, p. 18)

This book is about impairment of movement control which cannot be explained on the basis of disruptions to afferent and/or efferent sensory-motor systems, poor or absent comprehension of the task in hand, intellectual deficit, inadequate attention or poor co-operation. It is about the person who, despite a full range of limb movements, is nevertheless unable to carry out, under all or certain circumstances, actions which they previously were able to execute; or the individual who displays degrees and types of movement dysfunction beyond what would be expected on the basis of recognisable motor, sensory, language, intellectual or interactional deficits. Both acquired and developmental forms have been described. It is not a rare sequel of brain damage.

Dyspraxia occurred in 50 per cent of unpreselected left brain-damaged patients reviewed by De Renzi, Motti and Nichelli (1980). De Ajuriaguerra, Hécaen and Angelergues (1960) found constructional dyspraxia in over 60 per cent of their right brain-damaged group. De Renzi, Pieczuro and Vignolo (1966) found 80 per cent of dysphasics to be also dyspraxic.

Despite this, a perusal of the major medical and clinical textbooks, even specialist ones on neurology, movement disorders, strokes and head injury, will probably be rewarded with only a cursory and distorted — possibly even inaccurate — mention of dyspraxia. Sometimes there may be a few pages on the subject. Discussions beyond that are very rare.

Benson (1979, p. 172) notes that dyspraxia is 'one of the most consistently misused terms in medical literature'. Nursing textbooks hardly ever mention the disorder; paramedical works on physiotherapy, occupational therapy, speech pathology and rehabilitation in general, barely acknowledge the existence of dyspraxia, apart from perhaps one particular manifestation closely related to the work of the discipline

1

concerned. Seldom is there an accompanying discussion of the place of that dyspraxia within the overall framework of dyspraxias and movement disorders. Some clinical neuropsychology volumes offer greater detail but, in spite of the clinical label, might be too theoretically orientated for most clinicians. Many helpful articles exist in the specialist journals, but these are scattered.

One of the aims of this book is to draw together these disparate strands under one cover and go some way towards rectifying the imbalance in the attention paid to dyspraxia, especially in respect of the front-line clinical and rehabilitational problems posed by the disorder.

Why should dyspraxia have been so neglected and misunderstood clinically? It is not because dyspraxics turn up only in elite, highly equipped and specialist centres, which one might be led to believe from much of the literature. Dyspraxics are not found only in neurology and neurosurgical units, but in general medical and surgical wards, geriatric units, outpatient clinics, nursing homes and in community practices.

Neither is it because the disorder is never a severely handicapping condition. It might not be an acute, life-threatening state, but for many people it represents the main hurdle back to an independent and fulfilling life after brain injury.

Dyspraxia is easy to overlook. Its symptoms can be passed over easily and misguidedly as resulting from other more obvious difficulties, such as hemiplegia, use of a non-preferred hand, visual field defects, dysphasia or suspected dementia. Some dyspraxics have an associated anosognosia and so they do not report difficulties; they may even deny having any problems at all.

But worse than simply missing dyspraxic symptoms is that their non-appreciation and non-recognition easily leads to misdiagnoses and consequent mismanagement of the patient. It has been known for some dyspraxics to have been falsely labelled as being confused, demented, mentally retarded, malingerers and as psychiatric cases. The dire effect this can have on an already puzzled and depressed person is obvious.

At best, such people would be left in their frustration with the explanation that it is just 'part of the general upset to the system', or 'there is bound to be a bit of clumsiness using a hand you're not used to', or, 'none of us is getting any younger, and we all get mixed up sometimes'. Worse, they might be treated as simpletons, consigned wrongly to continuing care, put on needless drug regimes for their alleged psychiatric state and denied proper help so that they never regain their rightful place in society.

Dyspraxia is easy to be missed where assessment favours a meter-reading approach. It will not show up in cerebrospinal fluid analyses, muscle biopsies or routine central nervous system (CNS) observations. Neither, by its very definition (see below), will it be disclosed by examination of reflexes, muscle power and tone, primary sensation or cranial nerve function.

Dyspraxia will usually only be recognised through informed observation or by administering specific assessments. These tend not to be routinely and systematically carried out. Furthermore, in identifying, describing and 'quantifying' the difference between normal and abnormal movement patterns in general, and dyspraxia in particular, the examiner does not have available the same highly codified parameters of measurement as, for example, in the quantifications of trace elements, respiratory function or, more comparably, descriptions of language and communication applied in examining for dysphasia. Again, it is hoped that this book will go some way towards providing enlightenment in this field.

The main weight of the book's discussion will be towards practical aspects, and for this reason theoretical matters are kept to a minimum. This is not to relegate theory of dyspraxia to a subsidiary level. In the search for causes, neurophysiological correlates of the behavioural manifestations and hence a clinically and rehabilitationally useful classification and explanation, there still remain many questions of theory that are disputed or undiscovered. Where controversy exists these are mentioned, as are some of the more central theoretical considerations. References are inserted at the relevant junctures for those wishing to pursue matters of theory.

Two matters prerequisite to the detailed discussion of the dyspraxias, and which closely link theory and practice, are their definition and classification.

Defining Dyspraxia

Classically, dyspraxia is defined as a disturbance in the programming and execution of learned, volitional, purposeful movement, in the presence of normal reflexes, power, tone, co-ordination and sensation, and in the absence of visual, auditory, language, attentional and intellectual disturbances. Where there is dysfunction in any of these areas, they are insufficient to account for either the degree or nature of the errors found. With some modifications, explained in the main chapters, this is the view adopted in this book.

The literature speaks of both *a*praxia and *dys*praxia. Strictly speaking, apraxia denotes the complete absence of conscious, purposeful movement, whereas dyspraxia means some degree of malfunction between complete absence and normal movement. Unless specifically stated the two words are used in this book interchangeably, although dyspraxia is preferred as the discussion is about disrupted rather than absent movement. The corresponding words for normal action and intact intentional movement are praxis and eupraxis.

The above definition has several implications that aid the understanding, assessment and treatment of dyspraxia, and which are now expanded.

A Disorder of the CNS

As such, dyspraxia is contrasted with peripheral neuropathies and myopathies, that is, disorders involving the lower motor neuron, the neuromuscular junction and muscle function. It also contrasts with orthopaedic movement difficulties. While this may not pose problems of differential diagnosis in adults, the picture may be more clouded in the infant or child.

A Higher Cortical Dysfunction

The classical view of dyspraxia is of a disorder of the higher cortical mental processes involved in the planning and execution of actions. While this is essentially true, some extension is necessary in the light of recent findings.

Patients have been described with circumscribed subcortical lesions (usually thalamic or striatal — see Chapters 2, 3, 4 and 6) resulting in dyspraxia. Also, some dyspraxias derive not from damage to specific cortical areas, but to subcortical connecting fibres. Further, there are disorders linked with subcortical dysfunctions that are close in nature to dyspraxia (see in particular Chapter 7).

As a higher cortical movement disorder, dyspraxia is distinguished from subcortical movement disorders, such as the disco-ordination of ataxia, the absence or slowness of movement in akinesia and bradykinesia, abnormal tone and postural reflexes, and abnormal vestibular functioning.

As a higher cortical dysfunction, the disorder in dyspraxia lies (in cognitive psychological terms) in the disruption to underlying processes. The disorder does not lie in individual behaviours. Thus, while in empirical terms it might be feasible to speak of the 'dyspraxia of pouring a cup of tea' or 'dyspraxia of waving goodbye' and, as some people do, 'dressing dyspraxia' (see Chapter 6), it is presumed here that these are behavioural manifestations of a more general underlying disability.

A Motor Disorder

As a disorder of motor planning and control, dyspraxia is separate from disruptions to action performance of a perceptual, afferent origin. Thus, in pure dyspraxia it should be demonstrated that there is normal tactile, kinaesthetic and proprioceptive input and unimpaired visual acuity.

Disorders of visual perception can feature in the differential diagnosis, as can factors such as hemispatial neglect, disorders of spatial exploration and disorders of orientation to corporeal and extra-corporeal space generally. A person who is unaware of the whereabouts of their body parts will be unable to locate or move them normally to command. In their attempts at purposeful movement, they will show corresponding disorganisation. A person with visual agnosia will not be able to locate objects to command, nor demonstrate their use. People with disorientation in space will have difficulty in copying geometrical figures and ordering objects and their component parts.

The patient with hemi-inattention will show difficulty with dressing, reading and writing, and will trip up or knock things over. The individual who has impaired haptics will not know if their glasses are on straight, if their teeth are in properly or if their bra is fastened correctly. All these behaviours can be caused by dyspraxia also, so the importance of accurate differential diagnosis is stressed to ensure the right intervention is implemented.

There is no afferent or perceptual dysfunction in pure forms of dyspraxia. However, the co-occurrence of dyspraxia with primary sensory and perceptual dysfunction is common. This renders more complicated decisions in differential diagnosis since there is more to it than simply establishing whether or not the disorder is only perceptual or only motor. The question is more likely to centre on what proportion these aspects of dysfunction are contributing to the person's disability.

Afferent and perceptual functions are extremely close to praxic functioning in that praxis is acquired largely through sensory channels, and ongoing activity takes place in a visual–spatial and tactile–kinaesthetic world that requires constant monitoring and feedback for adjustment of motor planning. This interdependence of sensory and motor components in acquisition and control of actions has been expressed by many in the use of alternate labels, such as apractognosia or sensory-motor dysfunction.

A Disorder of Voluntary Purposeful Action

The contrast here is with automatic, reflexive, random, non-purposive movement. This constitutes a main reason why dyspraxia is not recognised unless specifically sought by watching and asking the person to perform voluntary purposeful acts. It also indicates a criterion for confirming dyspraxia, that is, that a movement not performed at one time be correctly carried out in another instance.

The person might be unable to smile, frown or laugh to command, and yet when observed in spontaneous situations they demonstrate normal facial expression. They might be unable to show how to scratch their head or touch their nose, and yet are seen to do so 'subconsciously' while watching TV or eating dinner. When asked to name what they are drinking, they may struggle to say the word *tea* without distortion of the sounds, and yet were heard to say it clearly when casually asked minutes earlier whether they wanted tea or coffee.

Further, they may perform each of the following normally — blinking to menace, turning the head to a sudden noise, staring around aimlessly while in thought — and yet none of them is possible under conscious control to command. Similarly, overlearned activities done without conscious consideration may be executed satisfactorily, but not when requested out of their normal context, or when only part acts are required. For instance, the smoker can strike a match while lighting up, but cannot demonstrate how to strike a match on its own, or light the gas instead of a cigarette. This feature of dyspraxia is also one that can lead to misdiagnosis of dysphasia, confusion, obstinacy, psychiatric disorder or dementia if the characteristic behaviours of dyspraxia are not recognised.

A Disorder with Specific Error Types

Dyspraxia is not diagnosed simply by exclusion of perceptual, language, subcortical motor or intellectual disorders. There are also errors of inclusion characteristic of disordered praxis. The derailments to the programming and execution of actions typical of the separate dyspraxias are discussed in Chapters 2 to 7.

Classification of the Dyspraxias

Dyspraxia is not a single, invariant pattern of breakdown of movement, any more than dysphasia labels one variety of language disorder, or agnosia or dysgnosia label one form of perceptual deficit. Dyspraxia is a general term for several qualitatively different forms of disruption. Signoret and North (1979) listed 31 types of alleged dyspraxia. Several more could be added and still not have exhausted the reports in the literature. Many taxonomies have been attempted, and variations stem from several sources.

As with any CNS dysfunction, description can take place on several different levels. Descriptions at different levels do not have to be mutually exclusive, though much argument has been generated in the past by workers confusing, for example, physical with psychological descriptions. Dyspraxia can be classified according to the following details.

Anatomical–Physiological Arrangements

In anatomical–physiological discussion, dyspraxia has been one of the many areas where the holist–localisationist argument has been waged (compare Geschwind, 1965; Brown, 1972, 1977; Luria, 1973; Heilman, Rothi and Valenstein, 1982). Geschwind (1965) and others have spoken of dyspraxia as a disconnection syndrome. Others (for example, Luria, 1973) have emphasised a dynamic localisationist perspective.

Cognitive Psychological Processes

In cognitive psychological discussion, while some authors have considered multiple processes, others have focused on more specific areas. De Ajuriaguerra and Tissot (1969) concentrated on the spatial aspects of dyspraxic disruption. They saw ideomotor dyspraxia as a disruption to actions centred on the body; ideational dyspraxia as a breakdown in concrete action space; and constructional dyspraxia as a failure of actions in Euclidean space.

Kimura (1977, 1982); Roy (1982, 1983) and Roy and Square (1985) have drawn attention to dysfunctions of the temporal dimension in dyspraxia, that is absolute timing (onset and termination times), speed, ease of transition from one segment to the next, integrity of the sequential unfolding of the subparts of an action, and the perseveration of elements of one action into a later action (parapraxic errors). Another contrast often made within underlying cognitive processes is between conceptual programming dysfunction and executive processes.

Behavioural Accounts

These detail exactly what people with varying types of dyspraxia do when trying to carry out actions. Such accounts have also examined how behaviour varies under different stimulus and response conditions. Much is made in the assessment sections, later, of variable responses according to whether there is a verbal or gestural instruction, or whether real objects are used (see De Renzi, 1985).

Other authors have examined variations contingent upon the type of response to be made. For example, Hécaen and Rondot (1985) (see also Hécaen and Albert, 1978) consider it important whether the gesture demanded is symbolic, expressive, descriptive, arbitrary/meaningless, simple, complex, or with or without real objects. (See Chapter 2 for elaboration of these dimensions.)

Specific Activities Disrupted

Clinicians have isolated, on empirical grounds, domain-specific dyspraxias such as dressing or walking dyspraxia (see Chapter 6). It remains to be seen whether these divisions are justifiable on cognitive-psychological and anatomical-physiological grounds. To date, such conceptions have been criticised because: they assume that a unique set of motor processes can exist for one action separately from another; and because by concentrating on discrete behaviours one misses the ways in which movements are disrupted across the board and not just in the area of prime attention.

Spheres of Activity

Workers who contrast limb/gestural, proximal-distal, unilateral-bilateral, constructional, speech, and ocular motor dyspraxias use this 'spheres of activity' division. This book also adopts it because it is thought to be the taxonomy best suited to clinical matters.

Praxis should not be assumed to reside or be located exclusively at any single one of the above descriptive levels. Nor is it the simple summation of all these levels. It results from the concerted and simultaneous activity in all of them. As such, its nature goes beyond the plain addition of all the contributing parts. In their concerted working, a new function comes into being that qualitatively transcends the sophistication of movement or action that could be produced by any isolated dimension or straightforward addition.

In a unified description and explanation of dyspraxia one would be able to say that a person has difficulty with action X under conditions Y and Z. This difficulty could be codified in terms of the disruptions to the temporal and spatial co-ordinates of the movement. In turn, these could be explained with reference to specified breakdowns in recognised psychological processes involved in the formulation, evocation and/or execution of the movement. These breakdowns would be correlated to dysfunction in certain neurophysiological processes, which themselves may be related to structural anatomical failure.

As yet, no undisputed unified theory of praxis exists; thus any discussion of different dyspraxias will be arbitrary to some extent. In subsequent

Figure 1.1: Schematic Horizontal Section of Brain Showing Cortical–Cortical Association Fibres and Liepmann's Proposed Sites of Lesions Causing Different Dyspraxias

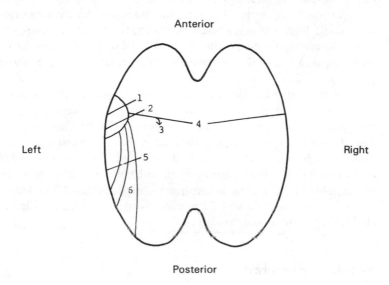

Key
1. Sympathetic dyspraxia (p. 37); 2. R. limb-kinetic dyspraxia (p. 40). L. ideomotor dyspraxia; 3. Lesion in the internal capsule; R. paresis, L. normal; 4. Callosal dyspraxia (Chapter 6); 5. R. and L. ideomotor dyspraxia from lesions of posterior-anterior association fibres; 6. More posterior or diffuse lesions believed by Liepmann to cause ideational dyspraxia.

chapters the descriptions given allude to all the listed dimensions, though the main emphasis is on clinical manifestations as related to performance in everyday activities.

Liepmann's Schema

The schema adopted here for the different dyspraxias is that derived from the work of Liepmann (1908) who was the first to attempt a unified view of dyspraxia as it is now known. Ocular-motor, constructional and developmental dyspraxias represent extensions of the concept to other areas since Liepmann's pioneering work. Liepmann conceived of dyspraxia in terms of disrupted psychological processes, which he linked to certain anatomical zones. He recognised:

1. An ideational dyspraxia, a disorder of gestural behaviour where the basic 'idea', or abstract planning process, was disrupted;

2. An ideomotor dyspraxia, resulting from a disconnection of the 'sensorium' in the left parietal lobe, where the planning supposedly took place, and the frontal zones of execution;

3. A limb-kinetic dyspraxia, which was the loss of 'kinetic memories' for a single limb and was caused by lesions to the motor cortex.

He also established the possibility of unilateral dyspraxias from lesions occurring at certain sites (see sympathetic dyspraxia, p. 37, and callosal dyspraxia, p. 28).

Apart from limb-kinetic dyspraxia (p. 40), Liepmann's formulations have stood the test of time, in that, currently, all workers speak of a conceptual and an executive aspect to dyspraxia. His strict associationist, diagram-maker, explanatory hypotheses, however, have undergone revision, through more recent models (Geschwind, 1965; Hrbek, 1977; Heilman and Rothi, 1985), especially those favouring a disconnectionist interpretation, remain close to Liepmann's original ideas. More detailed expositions and discussion of Liepmann's work can be found in Brown (1972) and Faglioni and Basso (1985).

Assessing for Dyspraxia

Discussion of the preliminaries in assessing brain-damaged people can be found in works dealing with the general issues (for example, Lezak, 1983; Filskov and Boll, 1981; Rosenthal *et al.*, 1983) and are not repeated here. Different dyspraxias are susceptible to disclosure through different angles and strategies of observation and assessment. These specifics are covered under the separate chapters. The following addresses aspects applicable to assessing all dyspraxias.

Methods and Aims of Assessment

Assessment is usually carried out and compared across several contrasting stimulus and response situations, for example, using verbal and gestural (imitation) instruction and with real objects. The latter condition can be subdivided into the use of objects in a test versus a naturalistic setting (on the ward, at home), in performing daily living tasks. Examination in different settings is important since success might vary considerably (Smith, 1979).

Measuring performance in naturalistic surroundings is also important in planning rehabilitation since, ultimately, this is where the person will have to succeed. It is also a well-known phenomenon that formal test results do not necessarily reflect functional capability. Newcombe and Ratcliff (1979) provide two particularly striking examples of this.

On occasions it may be necessary to assess performance to tactile stimulation only, or after passive manipulation of the person's limbs (p. 27). Reviews of the different dimensions and contents of dyspraxia testing are provided by Signoret and North (1979), De Renzi (1985) and throughout this book.

The aims of assessment are to establish the type and severity of dyspraxia and to differentiate dyspraxic disruptions to performance from those caused by other dysfunction — in particular, other movement disorders and language, visual–spatial, intellectual and neuropsychiatric impairment (Roberts, 1984).

Assessment must also describe the exact nature of the person's difficulty (for example, is it in recalling movements or organising different parts of a multi-stage action?) and how this affects his adjustment to the environment. The crucial aspect for remediation is not to tag on a label such as ideomotor or planning dyspraxia, but to find out when, in what ways and how far a person's ability breaks down. To say that someone is 'ideationally dyspraxic' represents only a starting point for help. It is only through the rigorous description of a person's behaviour that an accurate differential diagnosis will be arrived at, and a relevant, effective remedial programme devised.

Finer details of differential diagnosis and description of error types appear in other chapters. One issue that complicates and can easily distort evaluation of most dyspraxics is the presence of dysphasia. The converse is also true. Suggestions for circumventing this barrier to diagnosis are now made.

Comprehension Problems and Dyspraxia Assessment

In severe dysphasia, comprehension of pantomimed instructions may be better than verbal comprehension, especially in concrete situations, though this contention is not without controversy (Duffy and Watkins, 1984; Rothi and Heilman, 1985). Actions to be carried out can be indicated through pictures or by showing the objects that would be required for the activity. Complications that might arise with this method are discussed on pages 21 and 36. Goodglass and Kaplan (1983) provide an example and discussion of dysphasia assessment.

Reading comprehension might be superior to auditory input in some instances and instructions can be more easily conveyed in this manner. This is not routinely so, and cannot be assumed to provide a reliable alternative to spoken commands.

The role of observational assessment and reliance on qualitative error analysis becomes doubly important in severe dysphasia. Observation should be carried out by people knowledgeable about the manifestations of dyspraxia and who have more than passing contact with the person.

With milder cases the co-existence of dysphasia and dyspraxia presents a two-sided problem. How far are the person's poor (action) responses on comprehension tests caused by the dyspraxia? How far are poor responses on testing for dyspraxia due to poor comprehension? This necessitates finding comprehension items where action responses are minimised, and praxic tests where language input is carefully monitored.

Items requiring minimal motor responses include questions that demand only a yes/no response, or gross as opposed to fine motor performance. One can ask for instance: 'Is this a chair?' while pointing to a chair or a pillow; 'Can a dog fly?'; 'is your name . . .?' A nod or shake of the head can substitute for yes or no where spoken responses are impossible, but the examiner must remember that head movements can be impaired in dyspraxia. Pointing to cards with 'yes' and 'no' printed on them is another possibility.

Where comprehension testing involves pointing, it is best to employ items where successive directions for pointing are well differentiated in space. In that way, even if there is dyspraxia, the accuracy of the response should be discernible.

Dyspraxia rather than language loss might be suspected if there is a marked difference in results between fine and gross instructions and on repeated trials — provided language complexity is controlled across situations. Thus, dyspraxia might be responsible if the person scores well on pointing to objects around the room, but fails on pointing to body parts ('Show me the window' versus 'Show me your nose'), or closely placed objects and pictures. Similarly, dyspraxia could be the cause if the person scores poorly at body part pointing or object identification one morning, but well the next, and then poorly again on the third day. Where scores are uniformly low across trials, the likelihood is that severe dysphasia, or some other dysfunction, is responsible for the person's low performance.

Where the person is able to verbalise, comprehension can be checked by getting the person to repeat the question or to explain what he is to do before carrying out the task. It may be possible to have the person indicate the instruction he is meant to carry out from among a set of three or four alternatives. Some workers (for example, Heilman and Rothi, 1985) advocate asking the person to indicate from a selection of mimes when the examiner is doing the right action, before they make their own attempt.

Clearly, the differentiation of dysphasic from dyspraxic failure is a complex business and only the briefest points for consideration have been mentioned here. The differentiation should not be approached glibly or passed over lightly, and ideally should be carried out by someone specialised in the field. Others should be aware that the absence of a response, or a wrong response, is not an unequivocal indicator of dyspraxia.

Relationship Between Language and Praxis

There is another respect in which the relationship of language and praxis is important for the understanding of dyspraxia, that is, from the point of view of the theory of underlying mechanisms in the brain. It seems too much of a coincidence that language and praxis should not only be located in the same hemisphere of the brain, but also share similar regions and pathways within that (left) hemisphere. Do they also share the same cognitive processes and underlying mechanisms? Do they develop and break down in the same way? Is the relationship merely one of anatomical contiguity? Are praxis and language unrelated, as might be suggested by reports where there is double dissociation between the two (De Ajuriaguerra *et al.*, 1960a; Tognola and Vignolo, 1980; Kertesz, 1985)?

Unfortunately, there is insufficient room in this clinically oriented work to delve into this important area. The issues are mentioned in some later chapters, but for detailed discussion readers may wish to consult Kimura (1982); Lehmkuhl, Poeck and Willmes (1983); Duffy and Watkins (1984) and Kertesz (1985).

Motor Tests

Some clinicians have used general batteries that test for motor dysfunction in searching for dyspraxia, such as tests of manual dexterity, the Halstead-Reitan Battery (Boll, 1981), or versions of Luria's neuropsychological tests (Christensen, 1975; Golden, 1981). These tests have only limited value in diagnosing dyspraxia.

Dyspraxics may fail on tests of dexterity such as finger-tapping, turning screws, pegboard and strength of grip tests, as well as some of the perceptual tasks. However, performance on these does not (despite Heilman's finding, 1975) differentiate them from other brain-damaged people (Pieczuro and Vignolo, 1967; Kimura, 1977; De Renzi, Motti and Nichelli, 1980). It is on tests that make demands on higher order planning and execution that dyspraxics will stand out as qualitatively different from other brain-damaged patients.

Some of Luria's tests fulfil these requirements, for example, those of motor function. The 'Speech Regulation of the Motor Act' tests (Christensen, 1975, pp. 17–18) are especially sensitive in identifying what has been termed frontal, planning dyspraxia (p. 136). However, while Luria's test might help pick out dyspraxics, a detailed evaluation of the type and severity of dyspraxia requires closer qualitative understanding of error types. This information is offered in Chapters 2 to 7.

Although the batteries just mentioned may not be the most reliable or economical in identifying dyspraxia, the wider value of them in motor assessments is not denied.

Conclusion

The textbook definition of dyspraxia assumes the existence of an exclusively cortical, motor disruption of learned, voluntary and purposeful movement, which is not explained by other motor, sensory, language, intellectual or psychiatric disorders. The causes of brain damage do not respect textbook divisions, and so while patients are seen who fit the formal description, the identification of the dyspraxic element among a person's disordered behaviour is a more complex affair than the definition suggests.

In ontogeny the development of praxis is closely bound up with overall intellectual and cognitive development. Praxis emerges out of more primitive forms of movement. Acquisition of praxis is both a motor and a sensory process and, later on, language also becomes a regulating and planning force (see Chapter 7 for elaboration of these points). Ongoing action in the mature CNS also depends on intact higher cortical planning, feedback via sensory systems and properly functioning subcortical motor systems. Thus, it should come as no surprise that dyspraxia and its differential diagnosis are closely tied to intellectual, primary sensory-motor, perceptual and language (dys)function.

However, even though dyspraxia may be related to these other systems, it is not a primary motor-sensory disorder, nor a perceptual deficit, nor language-dependent, nor a defect due to disruption of motor control at lower, less elaborated levels of programming. While it may occur as part of a picture of general intellectual deterioration (dementia), it can occur with an otherwise normal intellect.

The multifactorial nature of praxic functioning also has implications for its understanding in anatomical–physiological and behavioural terms. There is no one 'centre' in the brain where praxis is located. It is the product of the concerted activity of multiple centres controlling multiple processes and utilising multiple pathways.

In turn, interruption to a part of this wide system will produce different types of derailments to action planning and execution, according to which part is affected. This will be shown in the different types of functional impairment and the varying quality of errors in response to different types of test.

Because dyspraxic behaviour might easily be mistaken for other disorders, careful attention to observation and the carrying out of tests sensitive to disclosing dyspraxic dysfunction is recommended. The methods for this are the subject of Chapters 2 to 7. Chapter 8 tackles the treatment of dyspraxic dysfunction.

One precondition for effective rehabilitation is the rigorous description and measurement of the dyspraxia, to which this book now turns.

2   THE GESTURAL DYSPRAXIAS

I was lying in bed and needed the nurse . . . All of a sudden I remembered you can beckon to someone and so I tried to beckon to the nurse — that is, move my left hand lightly back and forth. But she walked right past and paid no attention to my gesturing. I realised then that I'd completely forgotten how to beckon to someone. It appeared I'd even forgotten how to gesture with my hands so that someone could understand what I meant.

L. Zasetsky (Luria, 1972, p. 49)

Traditionally, discussion of dyspraxia has centred around disruptions to volitional limb movement, whether this has been in response to instructions to (re)produce arbitrary, meaningless postures; meaningful, conventional gestures; or in handling objects. For many, gestural dyspraxias are the only true dyspraxias, the others being seen as disturbances due to other reasons, such as dysfunction in other aspects involved in motor planning (for example, visual-perceptual), defects in different symbol systems (for example, linguistic), or in other motor systems (such as ocular-motor or extrapyramidal).

There are several assumptions implicit in grouping ideational, ideomotor and oral dyspraxia under the collective heading of gestural dyspraxias. First, there is the implication that the disorders described represent breakdowns to one type of action planning, albeit at different stages in its realisation. Second, as a rider to this, is the assumption that gestural dyspraxias share particular error types. Where variations in error type are found, these are considered attributable to derailments at different planning *levels*, rather than in different planning systems. Third, as a sequel to this assumption, is the belief that if other types of dyspraxia *do* exist, then they must involve breakdown of volitional action planning in other areas. As such it is assumed that gestural dyspraxias can occur independent of the existence, or severity, of other dyspraxias, and that there will be qualitatively different errors between the different groupings. While this certainly holds regarding ocular-motor dyspraxia, and is relatively well substantiated for constructional dyspraxia (Chapter 3), there are strong arguments (see Chapter 4) for seeing commonalities in the error types of gestural and speech dyspraxias.

These assumptions have more than just theoretical and taxonomical import. Clinically, they will influence what one is looking for, how one

16

is to assess it and what intervention strategies one is to choose. The following sections discuss the so-called gestural, limb dyspraxias chiefly with these ends in mind. Some of the more central theoretical issues involved are highlighted nevertheless.

Ideational Dyspraxia

The caricature of the ideational dyspraxic, Signoret and North (1979) remarked, is the person who fails the inevitable lighting-the-candle-with-a-match test. They try to strike the candle against the box, then try to light the wrong end, and with an unlit match at that. Alternatively, they stick the candle in their mouth and light it like a cigarette; or they produce any one of many possible derailments of the overall act.

Describing Ideational Dyspraxia

There are several views on what constitutes ideational dyspraxia (see p. 23). The core behaviour accepted in this chapter as characterising it, is a breakdown of the ordering and relationship, one to another, of subcomponents in activities that require a sequence of activities to achieve the end, that is, a disability in carrying out complex sequential motor acts. It is particularly apparent when the use of multiple objects and transformations is required. There may be misuse of objects within the action.

'Complex' is to be understood relatively. The seemingly straightforward tasks of putting on a shoe, or turning on a tap may be complex for the ideational dyspraxic. One must not be misled, either, into thinking of sequential actions only as those that utilise several objects or require several transformations of one object, for example, grilling toast or opening a door. Even putting up a hand to an ear, or taking the potato from a plate to a mouth demands a succession of actions, even though their separation is not as apparent as the stages in making a cup of tea or tying a lace. However, it is in actions using multiple objects that this type of dyspraxia is most clearly seen.

In pure ideational dyspraxia (that is, no element of ideomotor dyspraxia), the individual segments of the action are effortlessly and fluently carried out. This is in contrast to the clumsy, laborious and dysfluent way in which ideomotor dyspraxics execute actions. Also in contrast to ideomotor dyspraxia is performance on everyday activities. In general, ideomotor dyspraxics are only detected on specific testing, and they have little difficulty in performing familiar acts in familiar surroundings.

However, ideational dyspraxics stand out as abnormal even in their every-day, routine behaviour, though in mild cases it might be only on less familiar tasks or in less familiar surroundings that the abnormalities appear.

This description of ideational dyspraxia as a disruption in the con-ception rather than execution of the gesture is essentially that developed by Liepmann (1908) and co-workers in the early years of this century. The view is currently followed by Brown (1977), Poeck and Lehmkuhl (1980a, b) and Poeck (1983). The alternative perspectives on the disorder are outlined below.

Error Analysis

Certain errors characterise performance:

1. Elements occur in the wrong order. The person might pour water in the cup before putting tea in;

2. Sections of the sequence are omitted. The kettle is put on the stove with no water inside;

3. Two or more elements may be blended together. The person lifts sugar towards the cup, at the same time as making a stirring motion;

4. The action remains incomplete. Cutting their meat, such people take one slice at it and try to eat it, even though it has not been com-pletely cut;

5. The action overshoots what is necessary. Asked to take off their coat, the person proceeds to take off all their clothes. Instead of a drop of milk in the cup for the tea, they will fill the whole cup;

6. Objects are used inappropriately, either for the context, or overall wrongly. Instead of spooning sugar into the cup of tea, the person eats the sugar from the spoon. A pencil might be used as a comb. The candle is struck instead of the match;

7. Movements may be made in the wrong plane or wrong direction. The person might 'stir' their tea by lifting the spoon up and down. They might make a pulling-away motion when trying to push in a plug;

8. Many of these errors can be interpreted as perseveratory. After pouring the tea from the pot into the cup, the person might then perform a similar act with the sugar bowl, instead of spooning it in;

9. Many patients, in their endeavour to rectify what they realise is wrong, may make several abortive runs at a task before succeeding or, frustrated and non-plussed, giving up. These are reminiscent of the *con-duits d'approche* of some dysphasics trying to say a word correctly (see p. 106–7 for example).

These errors types represent descriptive categories. They do not explain *why* the person makes them. Just because ideational dyspraxics can be described as mistaking the correct plane for an action does not necessarily mean they have a visual–spatial disorder; just because they apparently misuse objects does not mean they do not recognise their function; and just because they make perseveratory errors does not indicate that ideational dyspraxia can be reduced to a perseveratory disorder.

Case Examples

The following include some personal cases and one from the literature, where many of these error types can be seen.

On the ward a continent patient was given the bottle in sufficient time, but nevertheless wet himself and the bed because of his disability in co-ordinating the actions of putting the bottle in position, opening his pyjamas, directing the penis into the urinal and only then releasing urine. Another person was observed attempting to pour himself a drink of con-centrated orange which had to be diluted with water. First, he tried to pour the orange from the bottle into his glass before he had unscrewed the top. Having checked himself, he then unscrewed the cap but was still holding the bottle in the horizontal pouring position causing him to lose a lot of the orange over himself and the table. After righting the bottle, still with some orange in it, he then hesitantly emptied it into the water jug instead of the glass.

A lady clearing the table after dinner put the plate of scraps into the fridge and the butter into the rubbish bin next to it. She realised she was doing this, but could not terminate the action. The same lady, who had been discharged from hospital to spend a trial period alone at home, final-ly had to accept supervised residential accommodation after potentially serious accidents lighting the gas-stove. On one occasion she had ap-parently lit the match, blown it out and only then switched on the gas, which she left going. Only the fortunate arrival of a neighbour prevented her either gassing herself or causing an explosion. The incident which convinced her and others that she was unable to safely look after herself happened when she turned on the gas, then filled the kettle and only then struck a match, resulting in a minor explosion that, luckily, caused her only bad shock.

Clearly, the potential for inflicting injury due to mismanaging actions or omitting stages is great. Machinery might be started before necessary safety precautions have been taken; objects other than the plug might be placed in the electric socket. For example, another lady — mobile and alert — was allowed into the ward kitchen to assist with cooking. At one stage she had correctly picked up the oven glove to take a tray out of the hot oven, but then tried to use her unprotected hand to lift the tray, and would have received burns had she not been restrained. Transferring her to what seemed a less dangerous task exposed further difficulties. She tried to take plates from the washer-up with a drying motion, then tried to dry the towel with the plate. Shortly afterwards she broke a plate when she performed the setting-on-the-shelf motion with her towel hand and went to accept another wet plate with the dry one still in the other hand: to take the wet plate she released her grasp on the dry one.

Poeck and Lehmkuhl (1980a) described several typical scenes of ideational dyspraxics. One patient was given a cup and saucer, spoon, tin of coffee, an immersion heater and a saucepan of water and asked to make a cup of coffee. He opened the tin and emptied the whole contents into the cup. Then he took the tin lid and lifted the cup up a bit. After a gesture from the examiner he managed to get the lid back on. He then took the saucepan and, even though the heater was pushed towards him at the same time, he instead filled the cup brim full with water. Next he took the heater in one hand and the plug in the other and hesitantly stuck the element into the full cup, whereupon he made turning movements with it to the right and left. Taking the element out, but still holding it over the cup, he picked up the spoon in his left hand, shook it a bit, put it down, transferred the heater back and forth from one hand to another, motioned towards the cup and hesitated. The examiner pushed the water towards him, which the patient took and poured over the heater, which was dirty with coffee. Finally, he lifted the spoon again but neither to get coffee, nor to stir. Readers will no doubt be able to quote similar errors from their personal experience. The significance of these normal 'slips of the hand' (analogous to slips of the tongue in spoonerisms — 'beggs and acon' for breakfast, and the 'carutomobile' industry) as a key to understanding the breakdown at the idea level of action planning in ideational dyspraxia has been considered by Reason (1979), Roy (1982) and MacKay (1985).

Assessment

Diagnosis of ideational dyspraxia takes place through observation of the person's behaviour and the analysis of their errors in comparison with those outlined above. Clinical procedures for eliciting the behaviours have also been devised.

Poeck and Lehmkuhl (1980a) and Lehmkuhl and Poeck (1981) chose their tests on the basis that ideational dyspraxia is most plainly manifest on serial actions with multiple objects. Poeck and Lehmkuhl presented sets of real objects associated with a particular everyday activity and requested the person to carry it out. Examples included the coffee-making mentioned above; a plate, knife, bread, jam and butter to make a sandwich; paper, hole puncher and ring file, with the object of making holes in the paper and filing it; a tin of food, tin opener, stirring spoon with a hole in the centre and a saucepan — the person has to open the tin, empty the contents into the pot and stir it; a boiled egg, egg cup, spoon and salt-cellar — the patient has to open the egg and eat it; and putting a note and coins into a purse.

It should be possible to devise any series of activities, ranging from short to long, and familiar to less familiar, with which it would be possible to elicit ideational dyspraxic errors. It is less the actual objects of the investigation that are important, rather than the nature of the errors made with them.

Lehmkuhl and Poeck (1981) found that ideational dyspraxics were impaired in sequential tasks even where the use of individual objects was not required. They used 10 sets of five to seven photographs depicting stages in familiar sequences, for example, brushing teeth, opening a wine bottle, making coffee, dressing, putting on shoes, making a sandwich, a tin-opening exercise (as above), telephoning, hanging a picture and a loose-leaf file exercise (as above).

The first picture in each sequence portrays all the objects necessary for the activity, and the person is made familiar with what is expected of them using this picture. They then organise the cards into the correct sequence, either doing this themselves or by indicating to the examiner. Lehmkuhl and Poeck found that people without ideational dyspraxia completed the tests without any problem, but those with ideational dyspraxia were hesitant and often were undecided about the order of pictures. The presence of ideomotor dyspraxia and the severity of dysphasia exercised no influence over performance.

Apart from proving an effective assessment technique, the results added support for two contentions regarding ideational dyspraxia. First, as the test did not involve direct object utilisation, failure could not be ascribed to agnosia of usage (see below). Second, it pointed to a breakdown not in the motor execution, but in the conception of the action plan.

As ideational dyspraxia always affects performance bilaterally there should be no significant difference between the right and left hand beyond that expected because of natural hand preference.

Some patients are unaware (of all) of their errors, others are painfully aware that they are not succeeding. The picture is not unlike jargon dysphasics, some of whom talk on without concern for their errors, while others struggle to produce well-formed utterances.

Because ideational dyspraxia is almost without exception accompanied by receptive language disturbance, it is essential to ascertain what level of verbal instruction the person can understand. Constant vigilance is required to ensure incorrect responses are not due to miscomprehension of instructions. Fortunately, the above assessment procedures lend themselves well to introduction by gesture, mime and pictorial or visual demonstration.

Incidence

Ideational dyspraxia does not appear to be a common phenomenon, particularly in its purer forms. De Ajuriaguerra *et al.* (1960a) found it in only 4.36 per cent of the left post-rolandic lesion patients surveyed by them, and in only two from 55 patients with bilateral lesions. De Renzi, Pieczuro and Vignolo (1968) established it in 28 per cent of their left brain-damaged group — though it must be remembered that they were using different defining criteria. Furthermore, their series included a disproportionate number of dysphasics, which may have skewed the figure.

It is probable that the occurrence is higher than De Ajuriaguerra *et al.* suggest. Most clinicians do not specifically look for it, neither do they analyse behaviour in a way that is likely to disclose it. Many ideational dyspraxics have almost certainly been falsely classified as demented, or low performance on tests has been put down to poor comprehension. As ideational dyspraxia commonly co-occurs with other dyspraxias (especially ideomotor), visual-spatial deficits, constructional dyspraxia, neglect, visual field deficits, optic ataxia, ocular-motor disorders, language problems, dyscalculia and so on, it is readily understandable how easy it is to overlook or misinterpret symptoms. Also it resolves relatively quickly after cerebrovascular accident (CVA) and, therefore, will be missed if not assessed for in the early stages of recovery. Its appearance is relatively late in neoplastic lesions.

Localisation

Ideational dyspraxia can arise as a result of diffuse damage to the cerebral hemispheres, but it is clear from other studies that it also results from focal lesions. These lie exclusively in the left hemisphere. In cases where right hemisphere lesions have been indicated, there has either been bilateral damage (the two cases of De Ajuriaguerra *et al.*, 1960, or the person has been left handed (case three of Poeck and Lehmkuhl, 1980a), who is the same person reported in Poeck and Lehmkuhl, 1980b). In the five verified unilateral lesions of De Ajuriaguerra *et al.* (1960), three were temporal, one parieto-temporal, and one parieto-occipital. All of De Renzi *et al.*'s (1968) ideational dyspraxics had left cerebral lesions. Poeck and Lehmkuhl's (1980a) cases had, respectively, an infarct of the left angular gyrus artery, an infarct of the left middle cerebral artery, a haemorrhage in the right (this woman is the left-hander) posterior part of the Sylvian fissure, and an ischaemic lesion in the watershed region between the left-middle cerebral artery and the anterior and posterior cerebral arteries. Other reports have pointed to involvement of the supramarginal and angular gyri (see Signoret and North, 1979). Moreover, contrary to earlier claims, the lesion does not have to be extensive, as was radiologically attested in the subjects of Poeck and Lehmkuhl (1980a, b).

What is Ideational Dyspraxia?

A disorder has been presented here that is discrete from other sequelae of brain damage and whose most marked features can be described as an impairment in carrying out action sequences involving multiple objects. However, it has been disputed in the past, whether ideational dyspraxia is (1) a discrete disorder, and (2) whether it is most accurately characterised as a breakdown in the conception of organisation of actions.

Agnosia of Object Utilisation

Morlaas (1928) advanced the concept of ideational dyspraxia as essentially an object usage agnosia. The patient is able to recognise objects — that is, there is no frank visual agnosia — but they have lost the idea of how to use them.

That ideational dyspraxia is not foremost a perceptual disorder is clear from the patient's ability to handle correctly single objects and simple sequences, recognise gross misuses by others, select the correct usage from a choice of demonstrations and verbalise how an object/action should be accomplished, even if they themselves cannot do it. The central errors in ideational dyspraxia arise not in the utilisation of single objects in isolation, but in the planning of more complex events.

Such a conception can also be criticised on anatomical–theoretical grounds. Agnosias are disturbances in individual senses. Object utilisation is a multisensory act and an isolated visual-tactile agnosia has never been recorded, and in terms of the lesion that would be required to produce it, is never likely to be.

Contemporarily, the agnosia of utilisation view is represented by De Renzi *et al.* (1968) and De Renzi, Faglioni and Sorgato (1982). The difference in view is reflected in their assessment techniques, which concentrate on single object usage, rather than multi-object, sequential acts. De Renzi *et al.* (1968) used a series of objects (hammer, toothbrush, scissors, revolver!, pencil rubber, lock and key, and candle and matchbox) for which the patient was asked by words and gestures to demonstrate the usage. Two points were given for an immediate correct response; one point was given for hesitant or protracted responses, with possible unsuccessful movements preceding the correct one, or when performance was conceptually correct, but movements were awkward or somewhat inaccurate. Any other reply received zero.

Heilman (1973) concentrated on the difficulty in evoking a whole action programme and eliciting the correct motor sequences in response to verbal instruction. His subjects were able to perform well to imitation and on actual object use. His patients were closer to the modality-specific dyspraxics described on page 36.

Is Ideational Dyspraxia Really Dementia?

Another opinion expressed has been that ideational dyspraxia is really only secondary to the general mental deterioration seen in dementia (Zangwill, 1960), and as such results from poor memory, defective attention, loss of association and general disorientation. For Denny-Brown (1958), among others, it results from a diffuse lesion affecting the propositional use of objects. De Ajuriaguerra, Muller and Tissot (1960b) likewise see a close connection between dementia and ideational dyspraxia. Their views appear some way supported by the survey of De Ajuriaguerra *et al.* (1960), in which nine of the 11 cases were associated with confusion. Certainly, ideational dyspraxic-type symptoms are found in dementia. However, in the same way that dysphasic and dysgnosic-like symptoms are part of dementia, it would be wrong to argue that it is the sole cause of them, and that they do not occur outside of confusion of generalised origin.

As was noted above, many cases of ideational dyspraxia may have been overlooked through lack of specific observation or testing, or ideational dyspraxics might have been labelled as demented because of their abnormal behaviour. There are ample reports of cases in the literature of ideational dyspraxia where there were no signs of dementia; for example, the four cases of Poeck and Lehmkuhl (1980a), cases eight and nine of Brown (1972), and the personal cases quoted in this chapter.

Thus, while ideational dyspraxia may arise as an early or late indicator of dementia, and dementia sufferers show ideational-type errors, the two are not causally related.

Is Ideational Merely Severe Ideomotor Dyspraxia?

Another line of thought views ideational as only a severe form of ideomotor dyspraxia (Roy, 1978, 1982). First, gestures are affected on command, then to imitation, and finally at the most basic level in the very use of objects.

De Renzi *et al.* (1968) failed to establish a quantitative relationship between ideational and ideomotor dyspraxia, which should have been possible if one represented only a difference in degree from the other. Many others have drawn attention to the qualitatively variant errors characteristic of the two disorders (Brown, 1972; Signoret and North, 1979; Poeck and Lehmkuhl, 1980a; Poeck, 1982; this chapter). The fact that surveys (De Ajuriaguerra *et al.*, 1960a) and case reports have described patients with ideational dyspraxia free from any signs of ideomotor dyspraxia (which should be present if they are related by degree), provides further testimony to their independence.

Brown (1972) underlines the misguidedness of labelling ideational as severe ideomotor dyspraxia, by contrasting it with the more obvious error of describing posterior dysphasias as merely deteriorated intermediate forms.

Conclusion

Further controlled studies are required to ascertain more precisely the frequency of occurrence and prognosis of ideational dyspraxia after brain damage. The 4 per cent found by De Ajuriaguerra *et al.* (1960) is believed to be an under-estimation. The figures of De Renzi *et al.* (1968) are not directly comparable due to their different defining criteria. It is hoped that the description offered above will aid in the recognition of the disorder and the avoidance of wrong labelling. It is further hoped that it will assist in isolating and documenting behaviours to be targeted in therapy.

Ideational and ideomotor dyspraxia have been contrasted in this chapter as separate types of gestural disorder, even though they do co-occur. The description of ideomotor dyspraxia is now turned to.

Ideomotor Dyspraxia

If ideational dyspraxia is taken as a disruption to the conceptual, high level organisation of a motor plan, then ideomotor dyspraxia can be described as a disruption at an intermediate level. In its pure form, unassociated with ideational dyspraxia, the overall schema of the intended act is preserved and plainly apparent. The disturbance is at the level of the individual segments of the sequence. In ideational dyspraxia the flow from segment to segment is described as fluent, and the action within a segment (such as striking a match, turning a key) is smooth. In contrast, performance of individual units and the transition from unit to unit in ideomotor dyspraxia can be characterised as clumsy, awkward, laboured and non-fluent. However, the disorder is not one of simply poor manual dexterity (Pieczuro and Vignolo, 1967; see De Renzi, 1985, for review).

The ideomotor dyspraxic does not stand out as disabled in everyday life. Ideomotor dyspraxia is disclosed generally only through specific testing. This constitutes another marked variation with ideational dyspraxia. In imitating single gestures, the ideational dyspraxic manages relatively well, but falls down on object use, especially with multiple objects. Such people are not helped by contextualisation. In contrast, the ideomotor dyspraxic fails in decontextualised or artificial situations, when there are no real objects to use. However, they perform normally with real objects and when carrying out an action in the normal course of events.

Presumably, action using an object narrows the range of possibilities for the intrusion of errors and aids in the comprehension of the task. Contextualisation may enable more basic subcortical or automatic contributions to be made to the effective running of the action, which would be less likely in the more novel activity of miming. Furthermore, the person proceeds in a famliar task at their own speed in natural settings, and the order of actions they perform is likely to form a logical sequence. By contrast, assessment switches rapidly from one fragmentary, and usually unfamiliar, act to another totally unrelated activity.

The effects of ideomotor dyspraxia are bilateral, with the exception of certain unilateral dyspraxias (see page 37 and 130). It involves upper as well as lower limbs, and in oral or facial dyspraxia involves movements there also (page 46). The bilateral nature may often be masked by a hemiplegia.

Assessment

The precise content of the examination is, to a certain extent, arbitrary and depends on the initiative of the examiner, what is familiar to the patient, and the patient's circumstances, that is, their level of consciousness, mobility, degree of language impairment and so on.

Nevertheless, the examination should be structured to elicit the distinguishng features of ideomotor dyspraxia and to cover those areas that divide it from other disorders. Traditionally, several distinctions have been made. Responses have been elicited by verbal command, to imitation, by the person miming the use of objects they can see but not touch, or touch but not see (De Renzi, Faglioni and Sorgato, 1982), and by real object utilisation. On occasions Signoret and North (1979) encouraged the person to reproduce a gesture after the examiner had passively manipulated the patient's limb(s) into position. Responses to imitation have normally been taken as sufficient for screening purposes. Testing through other channels is essential for detecting modality specific ideomotor dyspraxia (page 36).

There should be no differences between left and right limb performance, save for the effects of a hemiplegia or paresis. A sympathetic dyspraxia (page 37) should be suspected if there is good right but poor left-sided performance. Each side must be assessed separately to disclose this. The evaluation of oro-facial, axial and gait movements is discussed later.

A trend reflected across several studies is that performance to verbal command is poorer than to imitation, although it does not always reach significance (Ohigashi, Hamanaka, Ohashi *et al.*, 1980; Watamori, Itoh, Fukusaka *et al.*, 1981; Lehmkuhl, Poeck and Willmes, 1983). This is not directly related to severity of comprehension deficit, since patients with good understanding perform as poorly as those with impaired comprehension. Utilisation of real objects is always easiest; ideational dyspraxia or some other disorder must be suspected if it is not.

There have also been several distinctions made in the nature of stimuli employed. A major dichotomy has been between *meaningful and meaningless* gestures (see items below for examples throughout). Pieczuro and Vignolo (1967) found that meaningless gestures were imitated significantly worse than meaningful ones. This applied only to left brain-damaged people. Right-sided lesion patients performed normally. The authors postulated that novel actions that could not be associated with a learned act, and therefore demanded a higher and more conscious degree of motor control, were more susceptible to disruption in ideomotor dyspraxia than symbolic, meaningful gestures that were closely related to learned movements. This notion finds support from Heilman, Schwartz and Geschwind (1975); Kimura (1977); Roy (1981) and Rothi and Heilman (1985), who found ideomotor dyspraxics impaired in acquiring even relatively straightforward new motor skills. Lehmkuhl *et al.* (1983) did not find a significant difference between meaningful and meaningless item scores.

Towards v. Away from Self. This distinction has been included by some clinicians on the assumption that there is a differentiation in acquisition and execution of movements in personal and extrapersonal space, which in turn may be differentially affected in brain damage (Brown, 1972; Hécaen and Albert, 1978; Hécaen and Rondot, 1985). For De Ajuriaguerra and Tissot (1969) the direction in space of an action is a crucial factor in the diagnosis and understanding of different dyspraxias. Signoret and North (1979) found gestures performed towards the self more often disturbed than those away from the body. De Renzi (1985) is more sceptical concerning the importance of this division.

Transitive v. Intransitive. Transitive movements involve the use of objects, whereas intransitive movements express ideas and feelings: the latter are noticeably more impaired in ideomotor dyspraxia. The reverse is true for ideational dyspraxia. Hécaen and Albert (1978) and Hécaen and Rondot (1985) have subdivided intransitive gestures into symbolic (sign of the cross; salute) and expressive (menacing gestures; indicating a bad odour) gestures. It is unlikely that this is a significant distinction for diagnosing ideomotor dyspraxia.

Sequenced v. Isolated. Again, this distinction is of prime use in differentiating ideational and ideomotor dyspraxia. Ideational dyspraxics perform relatively ably in single, static exercises but break down on sequential acts. Ideomotor dyspraxics fail already on isolated movements. There does not appear to be a qualitative difference in their errors between isolated and sequenced movements (De Renzi, Motti and Nichelli, 1980).

However, certain evidence points to performance differences between parietal and frontal lesion patients (Kimura, 1982; De Renzi, Faglioni, Lodesani and Vecchi, 1983). Parietal patients in these studies were impaired on both isolated and sequenced tasks, but frontal patients on the multiple movements only. This data can be interpreted to suggest that the parietal lobe exercises an overall planning role for movements, while the (premotor) frontal lobe has predominantly an executive role.

Work by Heilman, Rothi and Valenstein (1982), Roy (1983) and Rothi and Heilman (1985) suggests that ideomotor dyspraxics may have a 'receptive' component to their disorder, which may in turn affect rehabilitation efforts, and therefore may need to be assessed in some cases. They found that these dyspraxics were well able to discriminate between right and wrong performances demonstrated by the examiner where there was a gross error, for example, when a screwdriver was used as a hammer, or when the hand was put on the head instead of saluting. However, they were impaired when requested to discriminate between clean performances and the types or errors they made themselves. They could not choose correctly between using a screwdriver properly and clumsily, or between the proper hand posture for cleaning the teeth, and body part as object posture. In Heilman *et al.*'s group (1982), only those with more posterior lesions failed, while those with non-fluent dysphasia and more anterior lesions could still discriminate. Some of their posterior lesion group could not discriminate between well-executed actions either.

The following suggestions for items in assessment merely reflect a selection of those commonly used, and do not exclude examiners using other instructions to better suit the person or situation. Full ideomotor dyspraxia batteries can be found in Pieczuro and Vignolo (1967); Brown (1972); Goodglass and Kaplan (1983); Signoret and North (1979); Lehmkuhl *et al.* (1983).

1. Arms

(a) One-handed, meaningful:

Comb your hair;
Drink a cup of tea;
Wave goodbye;
Hammer a nail;

Brush your clothes;
Shave/put on lipstick;
Turn doorknob and open door;
Threaten someone.

(b) One-handed, meaningless:

Back of hand flat on forehead;
Closed fist on ear;
Draw vertical circle in air with little finger;
'Walk' with middle and forefinger away from self;
Thumb extended, fingers flat (not clenched) on palm, open and close them;

Palm with fingers spread on chest;
Hold palm, with arm horizontal in front of face to self, then to examiner.

(c) Two-handed, meaningful:

Fingers in ears for loud noise;
Rub hands as if cold;
Thread a needle;
Put on gloves;

Fold arms;
Climb a rope;
Cut finger nails;
Play a drum, holding drumsticks.

(d) Two-handed, meaningless:

Cross arms over chest;
'Screw' forefinger in to back of other hand;

One hand on eye, one on opposite ear;
Fist on chest, palm over mouth;

Interlock thumbs and forefingers;
Interlock fingers, palm on back of other hand;

Thumbs on table, backs of hands together.

2. Foot/legs
Draw a W on the floor or end of bed;
Stub out a cigarette;
Wipe foot/feet on mat;
Shake a stiff leg;

Flick something away sideways with foot;
Draw a figure 8;
Beat time with foot.

3. Whole body
Boxer stance;
Turn round 180° to get something off a high shelf;
Step backwards/forwards;

Dig a hole;
Bow;
Turn over lying down.

A quantitative value can be obtained by awarding two points for a correct imitation, one point for partially correct (state the criteria), and no points for deviant responses (for example, Pieczuro and Vignolo, 1967). De Renzi, Motti and Nichelli (1980) gave the person three attempts at an item. Three points were awarded if it was correct on the first try; two points for two tries; one for three; and none for more attempts.

However, ideomotor dyspraxia is not confirmed on the basis of quantitative measures, but according to the characteristic parapraxias, that is, the partial derailments, which typify the disorder.

Error Analysis

Goodglass and Kaplan (1983) and Kerschensteiner and Poeck (1974) have described the typical error patterns of ideomotor dyspraxics. The latter work concerned oral dyspraxia only, but Lehmkuhl *et al.* (1983) confirmed the error patterns to be the same for limb movements. The errors are seen most clearly on gestural acts without objects.

Body Part as Object. Requested to pretend to clean their teeth, normal subjects, beyond childhood (page 168) respond as if they were holding a real toothbrush in their hand. Their grasp and orientation to the mouth differ only in the absence of the real object. However, ideomotor dyspraxics frequently substitute a body part for the missing object. Thus, a finger might be used as a toothbrush and rubbed against the teeth (Figure 2.1), or the hand used as a razor and rubbed over the face.

Figure 2.1: Body Part as Object. This and other figures in Chapter 2 ans 6 are drawings taken from video recordings of patients

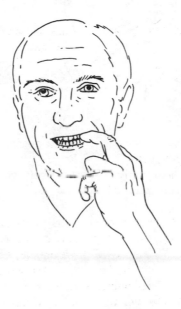

Altered Proximity. Normally, people pretending to carry out an action leave sufficient space for the absent object. Children to a certain age (page 168) and ideomotor dyspraxics may display a correct grasp, but perform the movement leaving no space for the pretend implement. For example, they will hold a closed fist before their mouth when pretending to clean the teeth (Figure 2.2), or stir with their hand in the imaginary tea, not above it.

Altered Plane. The correct movement or posture may be attained, but executed in the wrong plane. Asked to signal 'be quiet', the person may produce the suitable hand configuration, but place it and the arm in the wrong plane (Figure 2.3). The person in Figure 2.4 is holding the spoon in the wrong plane for stirring.

Fragmentary Responses. Asked to pretend that they are drinking a cup of tea, the person may bring the 'cup' to their mouth but not tilt it; in imitating a closed fist on the ear, they may complete only half of the item.

Figure 2.2: Altered Proximity

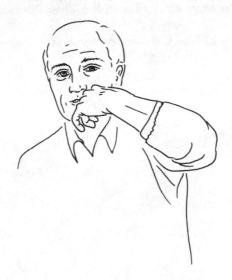

Figure 2.3: Altered Plane

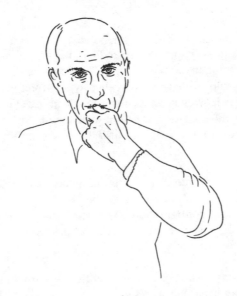

Figure 2.4: Altered Plane. Notice also the overlarge circle for the stirring movement, and the cross-palmar grasp

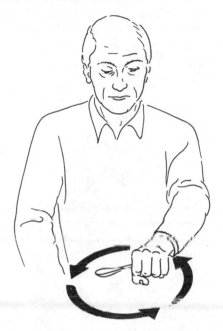

Reduced motivation, inattention, motor impersistence (page 13) and non-comprehension must be excluded as factors here.

Poor Distal Differentiation. Often, the overall arm position and plane are correct, but there is failure to produce accurate hand postures. Thus the person may give the correct posture for saluting but the palm, instead of being flat and with finger tips by the side of the head, is held in a neutral, undifferentiated manner (see pages 32 and 34). The man in Figure 2.5 is supposed to be smoking his pipe.

Gestural Enhancement. In this case responses are an augmentation of the actions required. While hammering, the person may show a synkinetic up-and-down motion of the head or a rocking back-and-forth of the whole body. On occasions, the additional body movement or facial expression may be the sole response for an action.

Vocal Overflow. This is a particular kind of gestural enhancement where additional noise accompanies or substitutes an action. There might be

Figure 2.5: Poor Distal Differentiation

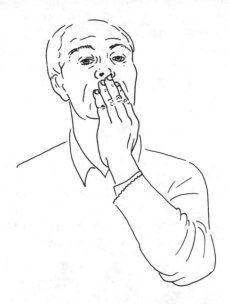

blowing or sucking noises when imitating how to smoke a cigarette. Other vocal overflow involves real words, such as 'hammer' or 'bang!' when demonstrating hammer use. Oral movements are especially susceptible to this kind of derailment (pages 48 and 54).

Pantomimed Context. This refers to a tendency or ability to be able to perform the correct action only when it is embedded in a lengthier act, usually corresponding to the context in which the gesture commonly occurs.

Perseveration. The perseverative errors of the ideomotor dyspraxic are notable. Kerschensteiner and Poeck (1974) and Lehmkuhl *et al.* (1983) found this category to be by far the most frequent error form. Perseveration was used by them not to signify perseveration of whole movements, but to refer to the retention of part features of a previous instruction in subsequent items. Not surprisingly, perseveratory tendency shows itself most strongly in the immediately succeeding items, but not uncommonly may appear up to 10 tasks later.

Perseveration of movement as well as of static postures can be seen. When requested to show how to shave or put on lipstick after having just performed a hammering exercise, the person may correctly put a hand to the mouth or face, but will hammer instead of performing a smooth movement.

Another type of perseveratory error is the substitution by, or accompaniment of, an action with older or more automatic movements. In these instances, perseveration is not so much from previous test items, but previously overlearned acts. Directed to touch the nose with a finger tip, the person's response might be to pinch the nose as if he was blowing it. A linguistic parallel to this is the tendency to imitate nonsense syllables as words they closely resemble.

Manipulation of Body Part. Lehmkuhl *et al.* (1983) classify this as a type of additional movement or gestural enhancement. In these cases the person tries to push or pull the body part concerned into the correct position. It happens particularly with oral–facial movements, but can be seen with arm and hand postures. For example, when asked to stick out the tongue, the person may try and pull it out.

The impression might have been given that the above errors are found only singly. This is far from true and, more often than not, elements of several error types can be discerned. In a personal case, a man was asked to show how he would clean his teeth. He gained the correct motion for brushing, but was using his forefinger as an object and performed the task on his head instead of at his mouth. The previous instruction had been, 'Show how you comb your hair', and his response had been merely to tap his closed hand on his head.

If ideomotor dyspraxia is not a crippling disability in the way that other dyspraxias can be, one might question whether it is worth the effort of the examiner and inconvenience to the patient to assess for it. Certain factors would appear to justify at least screening for it, even if a detailed test is left out.

Even though ideomotor dyspraxia does not prevent the carrying out of everyday activities, it does produce an awkwardness, clumsiness and intrusion of errors, which the person and his relatives may ascribe initially to having to use the non-preferred hand. It could become a source of frustration, depression and conflict when they fail to improve significantly with time and practice, especially in matters important to them such as writing or fine finger control. Being made aware of the potential difficulties and understanding them at an early stage in order to forestall later problems constitutes an important aspect of patient counselling. Furthermore, ideomotor dyspraxia may prove a hindrance if rehabilitation involves in any way discriminating correct and nearly correct movements, or learning new motor behaviours (Heilman *et al.*, 1975; Roy, 1981; Rothi and Heilman, 1985).

An unrecognised ideomotor dyspraxia can also lead to false diagnoses elsewhere. Failure, hesitance in, or perseveration on pointing to correct objects or pictures, and poor responses on asking people to demonstrate actions can give a distorted view on the severity of dysphasia. Poor responses on pointing to body parts or assuming particular postures can mislead one to a false assignation of body image disorder, or broader visual–spatial dysfunction. The slowness and seeming carelessness accompanying actions may erroneously invite a designation of intellectual impairment and dementia. On occasions, ideomotor dyspraxia may be the only abnormal clinical finding and it is important to recognise its presence.

Modality Specific Dyspraxia

In most dyspraxics there is no significant difference between performance to verbal and gestural command. However, there are patients in whom there is marked contrast between responses to verbal and gestural stimuli and where it is legitimate to speak of modality specific dyspraxia.

Heilman (1973) described three patients, whom he labelled ideationally dyspraxic. They were able to perform faultlessly to imitation, but failed badly on verbal request. Assal and Regli (1980) described a woman who had no visual agnosia and no overall dysphasia but was unable to name objects or pictures presented visually, demonstrating so-called optic aphasia (Larrabee *et al.*, 1985). Symbolic, meaningful gestures were realised without trouble in their natural context. Imitation of gestures was slow and hesitant, but correct. Miming object use to verbal instruction was satisfactory with both left and right hands. Presented with objects that were named for her, she had no trouble demonstrating their use, but errors were marked (20 to 30 per cent success) if the same objects were put before her and not named. Success was higher when the objects were out of sight and only tactile stimulation used (60 to 70 per cent success). Errors were mainly of utilisation: for example, a toothbrush was used as a knife, a cup as a hammer; the key was brought obliquely towards the lock, the turning movement replaced by a to-and-fro gesture. Errors on sequential tasks were also apparent: matches were taken correctly from the box, then discarded, after which the candle was rubbed against the matches.

From memory, the woman was able to draw normally with either hand. Copying models was impaired, more with the right than left hand. Similar left hand superiority for stick and block designs existed. Assal and Regli (1980) felt it was legitimate here to speak of a 'modality specific dyspraxia'. Analogous to optic aphasia, they proposed the label 'optic apraxia' for when a person is unable to respond gesturally to visually presented material, despite intact performance to verbal command.

De Renzi, Faglioni and Sorgato (1982) tested patients' ability to panto-mime the use of objects in response to verbal command only, visual stimulus only, or tactile stimulus only (after handling an object while blindfolded). More people failed on the verbal and visual tasks than with the tactile, probably because of the closeness of handling to real object use. However, there were dyspraxics who scored significantly worse in the verbal, visual or tactile modality compared to the other two. These data support the contention that modality specific dyspraxia exists.

Sympathetic Dyspraxia

In his diagram (Figure 1.1) of localising lesions causing various dys-praxias, Liepmann indicated two sites that involved transcallosal fibres. One produced a callosal dyspraxia proper (Chapter 6), the other caused a so-called *sympathetic dyspraxia*. This results from a left frontal lesion which compromises pyramidal fibres from Brodmann's area 4 to the right limb(s), giving a right hemiplegia or paresis, but which also catches left–right intercortical fibres, or their origins in Brodmann's area 6. This disconnects the right frontal control areas for left arm/leg movement from left hemisphere motor association cortex. The typical picture then is of a right hemiplegia or paresis and a left limb ideomotor dyspraxia. A Broca's type dysphasia frequently co-occurs.

Localisation and Frequency

Classically, since Liepmann, the cortical areas linked with ideomotor dyspraxia have been the left supramarginal gyrus and its posterior ex-tension and the left motor association cortex, plus the subcortical pathways connecting them (arcuate fasciculus, subcortical region below the parietal operculum and subcortical connections between secondary and primary motor cortex).

This schema has received recent support from Geschwind (1965), Heilman *et al.* (1982), and Kertesz and Ferro (1984). The cases of De Ajuriaguerra *et al.* (1960a) also support this conception. Basso, Luzzatti

Figure 2.6a: Lateral View of Left Cerebral Hemisphere. 1. Superior temporal gyrus; 2. Insula — hidden below opercula; 3. Frontal operculum and Broca's area (inferior third frontal convolution); 4. Frontal eye fields (Brodmann's area 8); 5. Parietal–occipital eye fields (Brodmann's area 7); 6. Supramarginal gyrus; 7. Angular gyrus

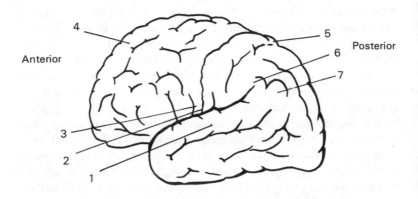

Figure 2.6b: Horizontal Section of Brain at Level of the Head of the Caudate Nucleus. 1. Frontal operculum; 2. Insula; 3. Temporal operculum; 4. Arcuate fasciculus

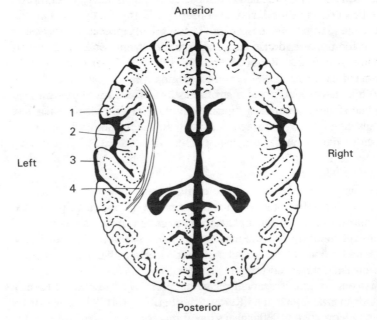

and Spinnler (1980) reviewed 123 left hemisphere brain scans after CVA. Their series did not contain any patients with frontal lesions. While broadly confirming classical notions of localisation, they found hardly any detectable difference between profiles for patients with and without dyspraxia, except for a higher frequency of deep-seated lesions in the non-dyspraxics. Neither did they find the volume of lesions a significant factor in the likelihood of occurrence of dyspraxia, its severity or its persistence. Furthermore, there were subjects with topographically equivalent lesions where one was dyspraxic and the other not, a finding common in research on many other higher cortical disorders. Agostoni, Coletti, Orlando *et al.* (1983) found cases of dyspraxics with lesions restricted to subcortical structures.

Clearly, one reason for the association of widespread areas of cortex and subcortex with ideomotor dyspraxia derives from the nature of dyspraxia as a disruption in the genesis and execution of an act that involves at least semantic conceptual, visual, kinaesthetic and motor contributions. More specific findings might have resulted if closer analysis had been made between stimulus mode, error type and lesion site. Basso *et al.* (1980) used only imitation of 10 single static gestures with a quantitative scoring system.

Brown's (1977) conceptualisation of the origins of actions would suggest the existence of qualitatively different pictures according to lesion site, a view that has been confirmed for oral dyspraxia. Lehmkuhl *et al.* (1983) did not identify any sub-types of ideomotor dyspraxia, but Kimura (1982), De Renzi (1985) and Roy and Square (1985) have presented evidence that suggests there might be.

While, not surprisingly, right hemisphere lesions have been reported associated with ideomotor dyspraxia in left-handers (see Poeck and Kerschensteiner (1971) for report and review), as well as bilateral lesions in right-handers (De Ajuriaguerra *et al.*, 1960), the co-occurrence of bilateral ideomotor dyspraxia with right-sided disruption in right-handers remains an area of contention.

De Ajuriaguerra *et al.* (1960a) reviewed possible instances, and De Renzi *et al.* (1980) were prompted to review the question after the results of their own investigations suggested that up to 20 per cent of their right brain-damaged people were ideomotor dyspraxics. Many of them were only mildly so, and the figure might be spuriously high as an artifact of their defining and scoring procedure. Nevertheless, there remained four (from 80 right brain-damaged) right-handers whose dyspraxia was so poor quantitatively and qualitatively as to be indistinguishable from that of clear-cut left hemisphere dyspraxics.

Considerable disparity exists between the recorded frequencies of ideomotor dyspraxia in brain damage. Discrepancies arise from sampling biases and definitions, testing and scoring variations. Poeck (1982) sets the figure at around 25 per cent; De Renzi *et al.* (1980) established it in 50 per cent of left-sided lesions; De Ajuriaguerra *et al.* (1960) found it in almost 19 per cent of their left lesioned group and in eight of 55 bilateral lesions. Within the major sub-types of ideomotor dyspraxia, that is, limb and oral, but excluding sympathetic and callosal, oral dyspraxia is the most frequent, occurring in up to 80 per cent of dysphasics, followed by upper limb deficit and, lastly, lower limb deficit.

Differential Diagnosis

The recognition of ideomotor dyspraxia may be confused with or clouded by several other commonly occurring or co-occurring sequelae of brain damage. Here the essential differences between them and ideomotor dyspraxia are discussed. Reference should be made to the works cited for a fuller consideration of the other dysfunctions themselves.

Limb-kinetic Dyspraxia

'Limb-kinetic dyspraxia' was the term used by Liepmann (1908) in his original formulations on dyspraxia to denote that dyspraxia arising from the loss of so-called kinetic memories for a single limb. The disorder, or ones very closely corresponding to it, has been discussed under numerous other labels (innervatory, motor, cortical motor pattern, melokinetic and kinetic dyspraxia). Recently, clinicians such as De Ajuriaguerra *et al.* (1969) and Kerschensteiner, Poeck and Lehmkuhl (1975) have excluded it from the true dyspraxias, seeing it at most as a disruption intermediate between dyspraxia and paresis. However, elements of it may be associated with ideomotor dyspraxia due to frontal lesions.

The predominant feature in limb-kinetic dyspraxia is a disruption of distal, fine movements, giving a slow, clumsy, coarse and even ataxic-like performance in which the target is always apparent. The sufferer is always aware of the difficulties. These features are invariable across stimulus modes, including the use of real objects. Furthermore, they are present in automatic as well as volitional acts. Difficulty increases in proportion to the degree of fine control demanded, not according to psychomotor complexity. Hence tasks such as writing, buttoning, sewing, playing musical instruments or making rapid, fine movements are impaired, while tasks that may pose problems for ideomotor or ideational dyspraxics, such as brushing the teeth or getting a cup of tea, are carried out essentially normally.

Limb-kinetic dyspraxia is unilateral, affecting the side opposite the lesion. The defect involves loss of movements rather than single muscles, for example, wrist extension or extension of some fingers. Tone and power are normal or only minimally disrupted. Sensation is always normal. Where there is involvement of the facial musculature, movements have been described as 'sloppy' (Brown, 1972), and the resultant fuzziness of speech articulation has been compared to the syndrome of phonetic disintegration. This is essentially a pyramidal movement disorder affecting distal parts of a limb rather than a dyspraxic disorder. It is seen as an isolated symptom of a minor cerebral lesion, at the onset of a progressive lesion in the premotor region, or as a residual after remission of a hemiplegia or hemiparesis. Where it co-exists with ideomotor dyspraxia, it may explain some of the clumsiness and awkwardness in transition between segments in a sequence, but it is not responsible for frank distortions and parapraxic errors.

Abnormal Reflex Activity

On occasions, the dyspraxic condition may be, to some extent, mimicked or complicated by the presence of abnormal reflex activity. The instinctive or forced grasp associated with frontal lesions anterior to Brodmann's areas 6 and 8, or the more true grasp reflex linked with lesions of those areas and of the cingulate gyrus, may be elicited on purposeful or incidental contact of the palm with objects (for example, the bed clothes, a cup of tea, their other hand) placed in it. The person may be unable to release voluntarily the grasp, though they might when their hand is empty. Attempts to pull the object from their hand increases the grasp, while pushing the object ulnar-wards tends to relax it. Stimulating the back of the palm may bring about reflex extension of the fingers and terminate the grasp. Abnormal grasp reflex may also be elicited as part of the general arm response on traction of the shoulder joint in lesions of rostral area 4.

Patients presenting with grasp reflex may follow or grope (hence sometimes called groping reflex) after the source of the stimulus. They may compulsively follow an object after it has been removed from their grasp. Such grasping or following may be elicited in the lips, giving a rooting response and pursuit movement of the head after a stimulus. Similar flexion can be seen in the foot.

Interference from overactive grasp reflexes has repercussions beyond actually holding objects. Denny-Brown (1958) describes the use of the hand as being overall clumsy, not opening far enough to take hold of objects, advancing too late and too far, and not being able to open and close quickly. The grasping overflows to produce stiffening of the whole limb. On passive manipulation, the patient may seem to be unduly resisting movement, which may be wrongly interpreted as intentional non-co-operation.

When endeavouring to write the person may seem unable to move the pencil, with the point apparently stuck hard to the paper: lines, if produced, are very heavy-handed. Attempts to walk produce stiffening of the involved leg as soon as pressure is exerted on it, causing it to be glued to the floor (see Chapter 6, gait dyspraxia). Denny-Brown included these phenomena as part of his syndrome of kinetic dyspraxia, terming it 'magnetic apraxia' because of the 'locked-on' nature of movements.

The converse to this he labelled 'repellent apraxia'. This is associated with the avoidance reactions released after parietal lobe lesion. Instead of contracting to tactile stimulation, the fingers extend — a reaction that may occur even on simply approaching a stimulus. When it is possible for the person to take hold of things, the grasp is light and the person may easily drop the object. This may affect the utilisation of objects: the pencil slips from the hand when trying to write; writing, if at all possible, is light and feathery, and the person appears to 'dither' above the paper and make only fleeting contacts.

Because of overextension, the person may be unable to insert the hand into a glove or the fingers into scissors or into the handle of a cup. The latter easily falls from the grasp if the person tries to take it with the whole hand. Avoidance reaction elicited at the mouth may cause turning away of the head and opening the mouth. Touching the arm may bring about its extension, making it seem as if the person is pushing the examiner away. A similar response might be produced when trying to introduce an object into the person's hand. These repellent movements are involuntary and not a sign of dislike of the tester. This does not necessarily mean that the patient *is not* fed-up by now of all of this assessment, of course.

The person who presents with abnormal grasping and avoidance reflexes may appear as if they do not have full control over their gestures, which indeed they do not. In contrast to the dyspraxic, though, the problem is not in planning the movement but in overcoming the interference from the reflexes. These occur irrespective of stimulus mode and are especially prominent in the handling of objects. The abnormal grasp can be distinguished in isolation from the postures of ideomotor and ideational dyspraxia by the following features: the thumb is fully extended at the inter-phalangeal joint and adducted, thus producing the main force of grasp between it and the index finger; performance is not facilitated by object use; the grasp increases with radial-ward pull and is released by ulnar-ward push.

'Utilisation behaviour' is a label used by Lhermitte (1983) to describe what he interprets as a more severe form of manual grasping behaviour. This is not reflex behaviour in the strict sense, since it involves higher level reactions. Tactile, visual–tactile or visual stimuli imply to the patient an order to grasp the objects and use them, without them being able to interrupt the sequence. The patient is subject to external visual and tactile stimuli in the same way as the patients described on p. 138 may be unable to suppress responses to auditory stimuli. Finding a plate and cutlery in the field of vision and reach, the person involuntarily begins to eat; seeing cigarettes and matches he automatically takes one out and lights up. The person reaches out to take things from the examiner, even though the latter does not signal this to happen, and even when displeasure is expressed at it occurring. The patient does not have to have some internal need, since he will grab food or drink despite just having finished a meal; or he may reach out for the urinal when the nurse returns with a fresh one, having only just used it. One of Lhermitte's patients ended up with three pairs of glasses on.

The behaviour is bilateral. It is associated with bifrontal lesions but it also arises with unilateral left or right lesions, still with bilateral effects.

Motor Impersistence

This refers to the inability of a patient to maintain a motor act, despite adequate comprehension and being able to attain the goal briefly, without any obvious difficulty. It occurs rarely in the normal aged person (Levin, 1973), but is found in brain-damaged people. It may result from cortical or some subcortical lesions (Cambier, Elghozi and Strube, 1980; Cambier, Graveleau, Decroix et al., 1983). Just how frequently it results varies from one study to another: Joynt, Benton and Fogel (1962) found 23 per cent; Ben-Yishay, Diller, Gerstman et al. (1968) 75 per cent; Levin (1973) 44 per cent. The figure may fluctuate because of different selection criteria. It is more prominent and persistent (up to months or years) in more severe neurological trauma, but in milder cases may be detectable only in the acute stage. The figure may also reflect different interpretations of the manifestations of impersistence.

Fisher (1956) included several characteristics. Impersistence in gaze behaviour prevented the person from being able to fix their gaze on an eccentric object, thus producing so-called ocular vacillation. This extended to difficulties in maintaining the eyes fixed on the examiner's face during, for example, visual field testing when the patient's gaze becomes attracted to the peripheral object.

Likewise, while assessing sensation or tactile localisation the person may be unable to keep the eyes shut, and the gaze is attracted to the point where he has been touched. The impersistence in eyelid closure may present difficulties for electro-encephalographic assessment if the subject is unable to keep the eyes closed on command.

Impersistence may complicate oral examination. The patient is incapable of holding open the mouth, keeping the tongue protruded, holding the breath, or sustaining vocalisation or exhalation. Assessment of hand grip may result in either a transitory squeeze or a series of intermittent grasps, rather than a maintained grasp. Similarly, in testing limb power the patient may only momentarily resist manipulation; and the individual may show poor persistence on tasks while testing co-ordination.

The contrast between dyspraxia and motor impersistence becomes blurred when one has to decide whether an action is incomplete because of an inability to plan and execute a whole programme, or because of incompleteness due to impersistence. The relationship between motor impersistence and dyspraxia is far from clear. There are ample cases of patients presenting with one but not the other disorder, but how far certain features claimed as dyspraxic manifestations may actually be motor impersistence is debatable. The status of alleged deficient responses is a case in point. If the patient, asked to salute, hesitantly raises the hand to the side of the head but then lets it drop again, is this an ideomotor dyspraxic error or motor impersistence? If a person requested to draw a house produces only the bare outline, is this constructional dyspraxia or motor impersistence?

There is no one formula that permits the immediate separation of symptoms. Decisions must be made in the context of the person's overall performance, both on formal testing and in daily living. Motor impersistence is mentioned here to draw awareness to it as a complicating factor in assessing the presence and severity of dyspraxia and as a possible added hurdle in rehabilitation (Ben-Yishay *et al.*, 1968).

Optic Ataxia

This is the impairment of hand movements performed under visual guidance towards a designated object or point, whether the stimulus is verbal or to imitation. In isolated lesions involving the superior parietal lobe it occurs in the presence of normal tone, power, coordination, sensation and in the absence of visual field defects, hemi-neglect, topographical disturbances, visual agnosias, dyspraxias and dysphasias. However, it is rare as an isolated symptom and seldom presents as the most prominent feature in multiple disabilities. It may co-occur with any of the above disorders in more widespread lesions. It is *not* rare in bilateral lesions of the posterior watershed regions.

Optic ataxia is most prominent in unilateral lesions when reaching under visual guidance with the hand contralateral to the lesion into the visual fields opposite the lesion (for example, the right hand into the right hemifields with a left-sided lesion). To a lesser degree, the difficulty is also apparent with either hand reaching into its contralateral visual field. Reaching under visual guidance with the hand ipsilateral to the lesion into the ipsilateral visual hemifield is normal (for example, in left-sided lesions with the left hand into the left visual fields). Misreaching tends to err medially to the target.

A striking difference, pathognomic of the disorder, is the stark contrast between reaching with and without visual guidance. For instance, the person cannot guide the hand into the armhole of a jacket held up for them to see, yet they will get the other or same arm in without bother if the jacket is held behind their back. Again, the patient has great difficulty when asked to touch the examiner's ear, eye or thumb in the affected field, and yet pointing to the same parts on his own body and without looking is performed faultlessly, in as far as there are no complicating factors.

Observationally, optic ataxia might be suspected when there is this contrast between visually and otherwise guided behaviour. The person has difficulty inserting keys in locks, pouring tea into cups, directing food on to a spoon or fork, and picking up objects efficiently. In the finger–nose test for ataxia, the person touches his own nose accurately enough, but may have marked problems locating the examiner's finger. Damasio and Benton (1979) described how their patient would typically undershoot in reaching and then advance under tactile guidance with her palm on the surface, giving the initial impression she was blind or partially sighted. However, she did not bump into objects or knock things down. The man reported by Auerbach and Alexander (1981) did bump into things to his left, and had unusual difficulty parking his car straight.

Contrasting with these behaviours, the person will button their shirt with ease and without looking, reach the light switch first time in the dark, and locate things accurately by sound or touch. For example, they will be able to indicate with one arm where they have been touched on the body, brush a fly off their arm, and pick a hair out of their eye or mouth.

Clinically, it can be simply demonstrated. Levine, Kaufman and Mohr (1978) used extensive testing, but Auerbach and Alexander (1981) found a modified simpler version sufficient. The patient was asked to fixate on the nose of the examiner. Then, using the index finger of a given hand, he was asked to touch the tip of a pencil held somewhere in front of him. Each hand was tested separately, reaching into both visual hemifields. The test was performed ably when no eye fixation was required, but with maintained central fixation, the errors increased according to the pattern described above. Perenin and Vighetto (1983) describe another procedure involving reaching the hand through a slit in a disc.

Discussion on differential diagnosis of optic ataxia and its possible underlying causes can be found in the works already quoted, and in Botez (1979), Megna, Bandiera, Nardulli *et al.* (1979) and De Renzi (1982). Hécaen and De Ajuriaguerra (1954) and De Renzi (1982) also discuss optic ataxia as part of Balint's syndrome.

Conclusion

Ideomotor dyspraxia has been discussed at some length, which may seem out of proportion to its clinical importance. This reflects partly its neglect hitherto as a disorder in its own right. While its effects are not dramatic, they are nevertheless a source of difficulties to patients, especially in the acquisition or relearning of skills. Hence, sympathetic and effective patient management demands it be recognised and acknowledged. Partly, too, the subject has been dealt with at length as it represents a complicating factor in many other disorders; certainly cases have occurred where patients have been thought to have other dysfunctions, whereas they were actually manifesting ideomotor dyspraxia. As a possible early presenting symptom of some progressive disorders, it is also important that its presence is not overlooked.

Oral-facial Dyspraxia

> They were overjoyed that I was home, threw their arms around me, and kissed me. But I wasn't able to kiss them — I had forgotten how.
>
> L. Zasetsky (Luria, 1972, p. 87)

Variously termed oral, facial, oro-facial, buccal, bucco-facial, non-verbal oral and lingual dyspraxia, this disorder can occur as a dyspraxia restricted to the oro-facial region, or as a feature of more general dyspraxia in which volitional oral and facial movements are also affected.

Apart from involving oro-facial praxis bilaterally, it can also involve voluntary coughing, blowing and conscious modification of breath stream patterns. Thus, not only may the person be impaired on oral-facial examination, but they may be incapable of producing voluntary coughs or deep breaths for the physiotherapist or during pulmonary function assessment; they may also be unable to close their eyes tightly or give a big smile when their facial tone and power is being checked. In addition, they may be unable to suck through a straw.

Assessment

As with limb praxic assessment, the actual instructions given reflect the discretion of the examiner and the circumstances of the patient. Instructions to verbal and imitative command should be included, as well as using real objects and/or observation in naturalistic settings. The tendency is for the patient to have most difficulty in following verbal instructions, then those given by imitation; while everyday real-life situations are the easiest to follow. Three broad types of commands have been used:

1. *Postural or elemental* settings involve the placement of the tongue or lips in a single, arbitrary position unassociated with any commonly performed activity. For example: protrude tongue beyond lips; touch top lip with tip of tongue; open mouth wide; bite bottom lip; round lips; and show teeth.

2. *Symbolic, co-ordinated* settings are still isolated movements, as opposed to sequential ones, but they demand the implementation of several sub-acts. For instance, whistling or kissing require settings of several parts of the vocal tract and modification of the breath stream: clear throat; kiss someone; gee-up a horse; blow out a match; chatter teeth; and blow out cheeks.

3. *Sequential* settings cover repetition of the same item several times, or strings of two or three separate items. Testing beyond three consecutive items begins to introduce too strong an element of memory capacity. Sequential tasks might involve blowing out the cheeks five times; or sticking out the tongue, showing the teeth or biting the bottom lip.

Observation in natural settings will establish whether the person exhibits normal, spontaneous facial expression (taking into account any facial weakness), licks his lips ably after eating and performs other actions spontaneously that he is unable to do to command.

Test batteries can be found in Moore, Rosenbek and La Pointe's report

(1976); Watamori *et al.* (1981); and Wertz, La Pointe and Rosenbek (1984). Despite the range of stimulus items and the number of subjects reported, there is remarkable agreement on the nature of errors found. Broadly, three categories can be discerned: substitutions; augmentations and additions, and deficient responses.

Error Analysis

Substitutions. These occur when an item is wholly replaced by another discrete movement. Asked to open and close the mouth, the person may open and close the eyes or protrude the tongue, or they might hold their mouth tightly to and nod their head forwards. Substitution may involve a distant body part. Asked to move the tongue laterally to either angle of the mouth, the person may swing a knee or hand from side to side.

Very typical of oral dyspraxia is the substitution of the correct response by a verbal label, especially with items involving modification of the air stream. Instead of clearing the throat the person may say 'Cough!' and simultaneously make a coughing gesture with the head or hand. Rather than produce the clicks to urge on a horse they may say 'Gee-up!' Occasionally, it may be a word unrelated to the instruction, such as 'Yes, yes'. Watamori *et al.* (1981) found different characteristics of sound intrusions according to dysphasia type. Their Broca II group (moderate to severe language impairment complicated by apraxia of speech), and to a lesser degree the Broca I group (mild language impairment accompanied by mild to severe apraxia of speech), peaked in noise substitutions that were of a fragmental, often undifferentiated form. Conduction and Wernicke's dysphasics, on the other hand, produced mainly onomatopoeic words: 'Puff, puff' for blowing; 'Hmm, hmm' for coughing. Other noises may substitute the desired response. The person might blow through an open mouth instead of showing his teeth.

Augmentation and Addition. This refers to the appearance of features, in addition to those requested, that are not part perseverations from previous items. For example, when patients protrude their tongues, they may at the same time nod their heads or close their eyes. Such synkinetic movements are a common phenomenon. Sometimes the additional movement may not be so closely related. The patient may wrinkle his forehead while rounding his lips. The additional gesture can appear in a distant body part as specific or amorphous associated movements of the limbs or trunk. The addition of extraneous or related noises or words provides a further clue to the presence of oral dyspraxia. When asked to round their lips, the person might also suck and/or blow, or call out 'Lips' or 'Yes'.

A feature which Kerschensteiner and Poeck (1974) include under additional movements with body parts, but which is classed separately by others, is the attempt to manipulate a body part with the hand. Occasionally, this might be seen in limb praxic assessment, but is much more common, though not invariably seen, in oral-facial testing. Asked to draw back the lips, the patient may try to push them back with their fingers; or they may try to pull their tongue from side to side.

Deficient Responses. These cover several not necessarily related phenomena. First, there may be no response, even though the examiner has established that the person can understand. There may be a marked delay in responding without any apparent activity, followed by a correct reply. Performance might be fragmentary, in that only a part of the instruction is carried out. For example, the tongue goes only to one corner of the mouth. The gesture may be correct overall, but not be executed in an ordinary manner. It is not unusual, for example, that, having been asked to show their teeth, the person will clench them tightly together and produce a marked grimace or exaggerated distortion of the face. Requested to chatter the teeth, the person may bang them together forcefully. There may be distortion of the range and rhythm of the movement as well as the force and velocity.

Trial and Error Groping. A visible struggle to achieve the desired positioning may be observed, and the successive tries are not necessarily systematically gradually nearer the target. The person may happen upon the configuration and then lose it. During the trial and error behaviour all the types of error mentioned above may intrude. Some subjects, depending on severity and awareness of errors, are able to self-correct.

Perseverations. By far the greatest percentage of derailments are parapraxic distortions with either tonic perseveration of a particular setting, or part perseverations. Part perseverations can be classified more realistically under substitutions and additions. Kerschensteiner and Poeck (1974) found perseveratory errors, in the sense of parapraxic part substitutions and augmentations, to be by far the commonest error type. They also established that elements of previous responses may contaminate subsequent attempts up to 12 items later, though the bulk of perseverations occurred in immediately succeeding tries.

Anterior dyspraxics are more typically associated with tonic perseveration, while more posterior lesions tend to be associated with parapraxic type perseveration. This point has been made by Brown (1977), supported by the data of Watamori *et al.* (1981) and others, expanded below in the discussion of the relationship of dyspraxia and dysphasic types.

It must be noted that while errors have been discussed as discrete entities, they do not necessarily occur separately. Any response may manifest features of several types. The patient in Figure 2.7, trying to put his tongue out, was at the same time breathing out and forcefully saying 'Huh!', opening and closing his eyes in opposition to opening and closing his mouth, while at the same time moving his head forwards.

Figure 2.7: Patient's Response Manifesting Features of Several Types. In trying to put out his tongue, the patient is also: breathing out with forceful utterances, opening and closing his eyes, and moving his head forwards

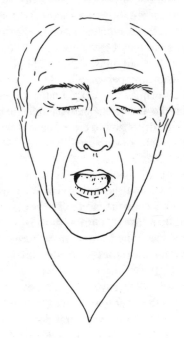

The predominance of amorphous responses claimed in earlier literature to characterise ideomotor or oral-facial dyspraxic replies does not appear to be upheld when the above taxonomy of errors is utilised. It is very seldom that one finds a response that does not fit into one of the categories.

The same classification can be used to analyse sequential responses, but added attention to derailments within the temporal unfolding is also required. One possible division is between fluent, normal speed utterances and an awkward, slow, non-fluent execution. It can be noted whether the person has difficulty switching from one position to another, and this can show itself in several ways.

In the most severe cases, provided there is a response, the person perseverates on the initial position, either not progressing beyond this or repeating it three times. In less severe cases, there may be varying degrees of contamination of subsequent positions by ones earlier in the sequence. Separation of the three items may be achieved in milder cases, but at the expense of fluency. Performance is slow and deliberate in such cases, possibly with a visible struggle to attain positions and gaps between sub-parts, such that in actual fact the sequence is produced as three distinct items rather than as a fluent, three-part sequence. Such awkwardness may only appear in the mildest cases if the patient is put under pressure to perform very quickly or to repeat the sequence over and over. Typically, it is the more anterior lesions that result in non-fluent execution.

Oral Dyspraxia and Dysphasia

One aspect of the debate about the relationship between dyspraxia and dysphasia (pp. 13 and 90) has been to ask how far oral dyspraxia correlates with speech pronunciation difficulties, and whether or not there are sub-types of (oral) dyspraxia corresponding to different dysphasic syndromes.

De Renzi, Pieczuro and Vignolo (1966) found oral dyspraxia in 90 per cent of Broca's (see Glossary), 83 per cent of phonemic jargon, 33 per cent of conduction dysphasics, and claimed it to be usually absent in Wernicke's dysphasics. They concluded that 'as a rule, the severity of oral apraxia is directly proportional to the severity of phonemic articulatory disturbances' (p. 69). However, their data permit an opposite interpretation, in that there were patients in whom speech performance was more severely impaired than non-verbal tasks, including four cases of severe speech disturbance with virtual absence of oral dyspraxia. They also had patients with oral dyspraxia but no pronunciation disorders.

So, while their conclusions 'as a rule' might reflect a tendency, this relationship cannot be interpreted as being of direct cause-and-effect because of the cases that clearly contradict this trend.

Kerschensteiner and Poeck (1974) found a correlation between the length of time a person had been dysphasic and the severity of oral dyspraxia, but did not find the gross type of dysphasia a critical factor in determining presence of dyspraxia. Overall, their Broca's group made the most errors in their response to verbal plus imitation commands, reflecting the trend in De Renzi *et al.*'s work (1966), which has been reproduced in all subsequent studies. However, their amnestic dysphasic group scored the most errors to verbal stimulus, with more than five times the errors of the imitation mode. The authors speculated that the difficulty of these patients 'evoking' a word or gesture might relate to a mutual underlying neuropsychological disturbance affecting realisation of a concept outside its natural context.

This hypothesis is confirmed to some extent by De Renzi *et al.* (1982), who found a definite sub-group among their dyspraxics where the central problem seemed one of evocation of movements. In the past, other writers have also discussed amnesic dyspraxia, seeing it as analogous to amnesic dysphasia (see Brown, 1972).

Kerschensteiner and Poeck (1974) supported De Renzi *et al.* (1982) in correlating the severity of oral dyspraxia and occurrence of phonemic paraphasias. Whether this was true for each individual subject is not stated. However, two other studies that concentrated on the analysis of misarticulation arrived at contrasting conclusions. La Pointe and Wertz (1974) found 'there was no relationship between the severity of a patient's articulatory deficit and his performance on isolated oral movement and oral-motor-sequencing tests' (p. 45). Bowman, Hodson and Simpson (1980) maintained their data did 'not support the conclusion that there is a relationship between the severity of oral apraxia and the severity of aphasic misarticulations' (p. 92).

A further observation supporting no direct link between oral dyspraxia and dysphasia is the variable rate at which the disorders resolve after CVA or head injury. One would expect them to improve in parallel if they were interdependent, and, similarly, deteriorate together in degenerative conditions.

Although data are conflicting regarding a direct correlation between oral dyspraxia and dysphasia (or, more narrowly, dysphasics' mispronunciations), another investigative line has pointed to a possible common underlying disruption. Mateer and Kimura (1977) tested groups of fluent and non-fluent dysphasics on isolated and sequential oral movements, both verbal and non-verbal. The non-fluent group performed by far the worst on the isolated movements, with no significant difference between all other groups. A different picture emerged on sequential tasks. This time the fluent dysphasics scored as badly as the non-fluent patients. Contrary to La Pointe and Wertz's (1974) conclusion, the problem did not appear to be one of sequencing: over 90 per cent of productions were in the correct order. Instead, errors seemed more of selection and omission, showing a failure to achieve target motor responses rather than just improper ordering.

From this evidence and subsequent studies (Mateer, 1978; Kimura, 1982), Kimura (1982) has suggested the existence of at least two systems in the control of speech/oral movements. One concerns the production of relatively discrete units; the second the smooth and orderly transition from one discrete unit to another. Anterior cortical zones were pointed to as subsuming isolated unit realisation and posterior zones for sequences.

Similar differentiation between fluent (posterior) and non-fluent (anterior) dysphasics on isolated and sequenced oral movements has been confirmed by Ohigashi *et al.* (1980) and Watamori *et al.* (1981).

Ohigashi *et al.*, like Mateer and Kimura (1977), found only the non-fluent group affected on isolated movements, a difference that disappeared when it came to sequential tasks. However, they were able to separate them by qualitative analysis, despite quantitative similarities in the error scores of the two groups on consecutive movements. The non-fluent group's difficulties on combined movements related back to the problems they had had with each of the movements individually on the isolated movements task. (Ohigashi *et al.*'s (1980) sequential tests consisted of only two items each.) In other words, their problem was a fundamental difficulty in the realisation of elementary oral gestures.

The fluent group, in contrast, made predominantly errors of transformation and seriation. Transformation means here the derailment of one of the elements in the sequenced gestures test, despite it having been correct in isolation. Seriation refers to reversal of the order of sub-items. Ohigashi *et al.*'s (1980) error analysis procedure is not as sensitive as it might be, but nevertheless points to an area of variation for further research.

Watamori *et al.* (1981) analysed errors in relation to stimulus type (verbal versus imitation), task demands (elemental versus co-ordinated, see p. 47) and dysphasia type. Like De Renzi *et al.* (1966) and Kerschensteiner and Poeck (1974), they found Broca's dysphasics most impaired on the praxis tests. They also corroborated Mateer and Kimura's (1977) anterior/non-fluent versus posterior/fluent distinction, though with some slight differences that they attributed to variation in test design. With a more detailed error analysis than Ohigashi *et al.* (1980), they found that error profiles yielded distinctly different pictures corresponding to each dysphasic group.

They found no significant variation between responses to verbal and imitation instructions for their two Broca's groups. The scores of their Wernicke's group to verbal command correlated with their comprehension scores, but they improved significantly to imitative command. The conduction dysphasics also achieved less well on verbal instruction, which was attributed by Watamori *et al.* (1981) to their poor comprehension of directions without any redundancy.

The four dysphasic groups also peaked on different error types. Their Broca I group (mild language impairment, mild to severe apraxia of speech) had a profile similar to that of normal people, but with marked delay in responses, which were accompanied by trial and error groping. The Broca II subjects (moderate to severe language impairment complicated by apraxia of speech) had a high percentage of 'no response' errors. Perseveration was a strong feature. The most characteristic derailments were 'noise' and 'additional noise' (p. 48). The noises were largely undifferentiated, fragmental sounds. The Wernicke's patients also had high noise and additional noise counts in the imitation tasks. Interestingly, in contrast to Broca II people, these were onomatopoeic sounds or words. The conduction group's errors resembled their phonological behaviour in speech, that is, frank substitutions and delays.

There is indication that the non-fluent/fluent or anterior/posterior distinction, and contrasts in error between delay, evocation, substitution and so on, is also found in limb and speech dyspraxia. Discussion concerning this is found in Brown (1977); Roy (1981); Kimura (1982); and in Chapter 4. Roy and Square (1985) have drawn together evidence from many sources in consideration of the argument. References for the wider relationship of dysphasia and dyspraxia are given in Chapter 1.

Localisation of Lesions Associated with Oral Dyspraxia

The localisation of lesions associated with facial/oral dyspraxia is similar to that for ideomotor dyspraxia. Geschwind (1965) mentions involvement of the supramarginal gyrus region, or fibres running from the posterial visual and auditory (speech) association areas via the arcuate fasciculus to anterior motor association areas. He attributes the finding of conduction dysphasia with facial but without limb dyspraxia, to the possible deeper course of fibres to facial pre-motor areas than fibres to limb areas. The finding of oral dyspraxia with posterior dysphasias supports a role of temporal–parietal regions in oral praxis.

In anterior lesions where association cortex anterior to the face area is destroyed, facial movements are impaired because of disconnection of the left face area from 'planning' areas and interruption of the origin of transcallosal fibres to the right facial regions. This is the classical view of Liepmann (1908) and the one advanced by Geschwind (1965).

Tognola and Vignolo (1980) reviewed the brain scans of patients with oral dyspraxia. They assessed praxis only with single movements and acknowledged that, in omitting sequential items, they perhaps did not capture all areas responsible in the genesis of voluntary oral movements. The chief areas implicated in their CVA patients (most of whom had dysphasia and dyspraxia, but some had dyspraxia only) were the frontal and central opercula, and a small area of the first temporal convolution, of the left hemisphere, in particular the anterior insula. This latter area might be prominent either because of its continuity with the overlying opercula, and/or because of damage to the insula also affecting the closely coursing temporo- and occipito-frontal fasciculi.

Conclusion

Oral-facial dyspraxia is found both as part of a general ideomotor dyspraxia and as an isolated oral-facial or oral dyspraxia. In their daily routine, like ideomotor dyspraxics, people with oral-facial dyspraxia do not generally stand out as being impaired. They have a normal facial expression, no chewing, swallowing or breathing difficulties, and need not necessarily have any speech difficulties. However, the recognition of oral-facial dyspraxia is important as it may bias assessment of other functions and be a complicating factor in therapy for apraxia of speech (Chapter 4). It is also a valuable area of investigation for studying the relationship of dyspraxia to dysphasia.

In behavioural terms, constructional dyspraxia (CD) is a disorder of planned movements for any kind of task involving the structuring or arranging of objects, parts of objects, or lines in two and three dimensional space. De Renzi (1982) emphasises the dual motor and visual–spatial aspects so important to an understanding of the disorder when he describes CD as 'emerging in the execution of tasks where individual elements must be arranged in a given spatial relationship to form a unitary structure, under the guidance of a visual or mental model' (p. 237).

Other writers have sought to capture the confluence of visual and motor processes with alternative labels, for example, visual–spatial agnosia (Brown, 1972), or apractognosia (Hécaen, Penfield, Bertrand et al., 1956).

Signoret and North (1979) and Hyvärinen (1982) (following Critchley) have drawn attention to the disruption of movement performed in extrapersonal space, the 'activity space' within the sphere of hands and fingers (Hyvärinen, p. 1076). Here, the difficulty emphasised is in changing the use of the limbs from a component of personal space into a tool or manipulator of 'tools', controlled in extrapersonal space.

A historical survey of the development of the concept of CD is provided by Warrington (1969) and De Renzi (1982). It is taken as understood that, as with all other dyspraxias, primary sensory and motor disruption has been excluded in defining CD.

Clinical Presentation

According to the degree of severity, CD might manifest itself in anything from a marked incapacitation on a whole range of everyday activities, to what might be reported as a mild 'confusion' or 'hamfistedness' in handling objects. In mild cases the underlying CD may only become apparent on specific tests. The picture can be further complicated by a number of commonly co-occurring dysfunctions (see below).

In the work situation, CD may result in an inability or impairment in using tools. This means not only obvious examples such as the tools of the carpenter or mechanic, but in the use of the hands or hand-controlled implements in any dismantling, assembly or manipulation job. The typist may no longer be able to change the ribbon or type head, put in the paper, or fold the letter in the envelope afterwards; the seamstress cannot change the thread; the packer cannot pack boxes or tie up knots; the draughtsman cannot draw correct lines, angles or diagrams; the builder cannot lay bricks or construct corners correctly; the person may no longer be able to write.

One personal case involved a woman very active in local government and a member of several committees. She suffered what subsequently was diagnosed as an embolic CVA, during or subsequent to a knee operation, but which at the time had passed unnoticed. Her language was unimpaired and at home she herself noticed only a mild confusion in dressing, tidying up and the like, which she attributed to the operation having 'taken it out of her at her age' (late sixties). Only on resuming her committee work did she realise that she had a genuine problem, since she found it impossible to write down the minutes.

A possible difficulty in differential diagnosis was highlighted in this case. Before her operation, the woman, who lived alone, had been very meticulous with her dress and the upkeep of her house. It was on the insistence of her relatives that she had sought medical advice as they claimed she was behaving peculiarly, and they suspected a psychiatric cause. The alleged peculiar behaviour related to the haphazard way in which she laid the table, with knives, forks and spoons scattered apparently at random in contrast to her previous strict attention to such decorum. The relatives had also noted that this previously immaculately dressed woman now appeared to dress herself in a slipshod manner and generally neglected her personal appearance. Their suspicions were increased by the patient's denial of any real difficulties. Observation of her writing and specific testing disclosed a clear case of CD associated with a right parietal CVA.

As this case illustrates, it is not only at work that CD may prove a handicap. Using kitchen utensils, assembling mixers, setting up the ironing board, actually doing the ironing and folding the clothes afterwards, have all been problems met in personal cases. Dressing may be affected (Chapter 6), thus making morning times a nightmare and shopping trips for clothes a chore.

Pastimes are not spared either. Tinkering with the car at weekends, cutting out patterns, numerous board games and many more activities become affected. During rehabilitation the person may experience difficulty learning to use certain aids as well as in primary target areas of housekeeping and occupational skills.

Clearly, the list of daily activities at risk is endless. The common underlying difficulty found in all is the inability to perceive how two or more parts relate to form a whole. Some patients may appreciate how the end product should be organised, but be unable to work out how the parts should be manipulated to achieve the aim. One patient was able to describe how the roll of film should be inserted into his camera, but when he actually tried, he could do no better than produce a series of apparently random juxtapositions of the two.

On occasions, the person's general behaviour clearly indicates CD, but usually specific testing will be necessary to confirm and quantify the diagnosis.

Assessment

Tests for CD fall into three main categories: observation in natural settings; semi-formal procedures; and formal batteries. The diversity and range of tests within these categories reflects the breadth of behaviours and situations that can be affected in CD. They also reflect a variety of theoretical standpoints regarding what CD is. The features one looks for in observational assessment are those covered in the clinical description and in the case histories mentioned in this chapter. The following tests deal with semi-formal and formal assessment. Several different types of assessment can be described.

Paper and Pencil Tests

These require the person to reproduce various figures either through tracing, by copying or from memory. Writing also falls within this section. Tasks range from the relatively straightforward copying of simple crosses (De Renzi and Faglioni, 1967), to reproduction of complex abstract designs such as the Rey-Osterrieth complex figure test (Osterrieth, 1944), or drawing from memory objects such as a flower, house, human figure or bike. Published tests include the Bender Gestalt test (Lacks, 1984), Benton visual retention test (Benton, 1974) and the Rey-Osterrieth figure (Osterreith, 1944). Warrington, James and Kinsbourne (1966) devised a set of structured and unstructured figures for use in their research.

Two-dimensional Construction

Block design and stick construction tests come under this category. Form boards, jig-saws and cardboard cut-out assembly are also essentially two-dimensional constructional tasks.

Goodglass and Kaplan (1983) provide examples of stick pattern tests. The examiner provides a model that the subject has to copy or reproduce from memory. Stick design can be tested without models by, for instance, asking the person to form a square or a W with their sticks (Figure 3.1).

Figure 3.1: Stick Design Performance by a Woman with a Right Parietal CVA. (a) Letters produced to verbal command; (b) models given to copy. Note dissolution of spatial relationships in (a), and rotation of copies in (b)

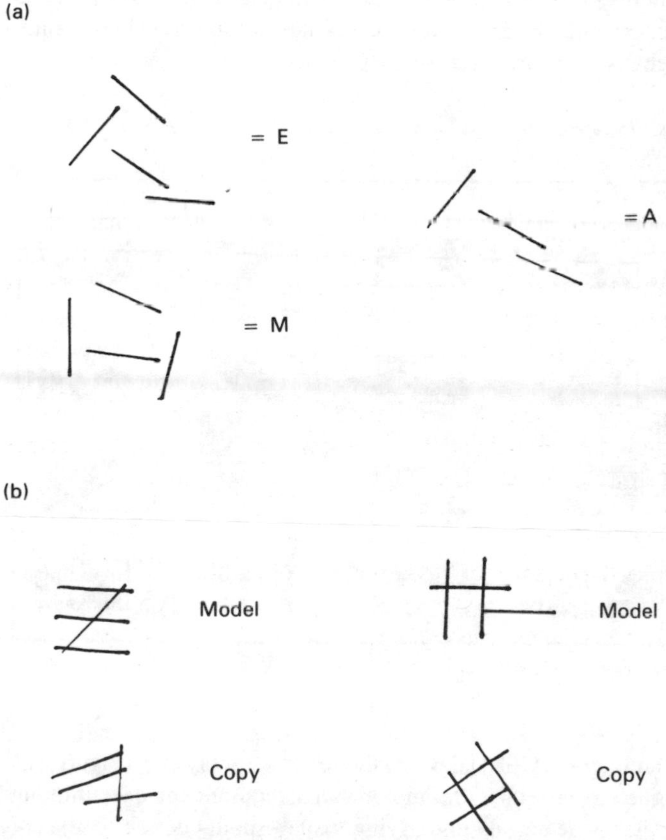

(a)

= E

= A

= M

(b)

Model

Model

Copy

Copy

The classical two-dimensional block design test is the Kohs block test or modifications of it in the Wechsler Adult Intelligence Scales (WAIS). Even though the blocks are three-dimensional, the patterns themselves are two-dimensional. While the block design section of the WAIS may suffice in most cases, the more difficult designs of the original Kohs test may help to detect mild constructional difficulties.

Consoli (1979) has devised a variation of the Kohs block test using 16 rectangles with various triangular patterns (Figure 3.2). The test discriminates well between constructional dyspraxics and normal people. It is also claimed to be useful in highlighting different strategies and error types typical of either right or left hemisphere CD. It further appears to be more sensitive than longer established tests, particularly for detecting left hemisphere CD. Consoli argues that this may be due to the minimal intervening language variables which are included in other tests and so penalise left brain-damaged patients.

Figure 3.2: Variation of the Kohs Block Test by Consoli (1979)

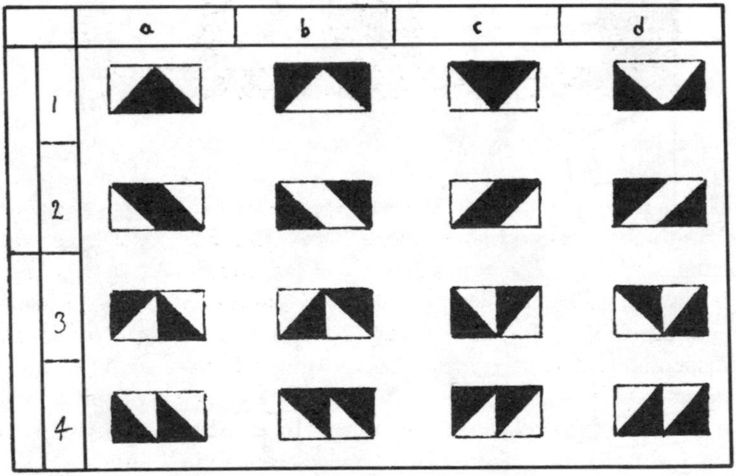

Source: Reproduced by courtesy of the editors, *Neuropsychologia*

Mack and Levine (1981) devised the form assembly task (Figure 3.3). It is designed to minimise the motor skills required for execution and therefore assess better any underlying visual–spatial deficit that is contributing to the constructional problem.

Three-dimensional Construction

Not only are three-dimensional tasks generally more difficult, but according to Benton and Fogel (1962), different skills and processes are being assessed in three-dimensional tests. Evaluation of performance in

Figure 3.3: The Form Assembly Task

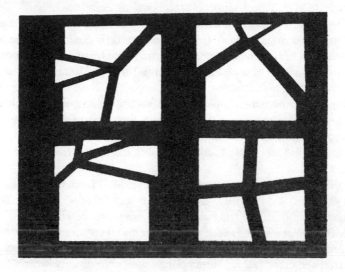

Source: Reproduced by courtesy of the editors, *Cortex*

this area involves three-dimensional object assembly tasks or the use of bricks to construct abstract designs. Benton and Fogel (1962) provide examples of these. Many more tests and procedures are available than it is possible to describe here. Lezak (1983) has reviewed many of them.

Alongside more formal tests, assessments on everyday activities are indispensable. After all, rehabilitation is aimed ultimately at enabling the person to resume normal daily living patterns, and not simply to raise the profile on this or that test. Assessment on daily living tasks may also give a different picture from that gained from formal tests.

The person may be able to perform the overlearned routines efficiently enough despite low scores on formal testing. Newcombe and Ratcliff (1979) provide particularly striking examples of this. The likelihood of efficient performance will be increased if the routines are carried out in familiar surroundings. While specialised tests may confirm that the person has CD and indicate why he is having difficulties, only assessment on natural activities will tell the therapist *what* specific problems are going to have to be dealt with in rehabilitation. This underlines the importance of description and qualitative evaluation of performance besides simply quantitative measures. With this, discussion has arrived at the question of how these measures are interpreted.

Interpretation of Results

The methods of assessment mentioned can be divided into those that give a numerical score and those that concentrate on a qualitative analysis. The division is somewhat artificial, in that quantitative scores are also based on counting deviations from normal that are assumed to be indicative of CD.

The individual tests mentioned detail their own scoring systems, and it is not possible to review them in depth here (see, for example, Arrigoni and De Renzi, 1964; De Renzi and Faglioni, 1967; Consoli, 1979; Mack and Levine, 1981; Lacks, 1984). Some of the features marked cover:

1. The strategy used in reproducing the model. Does the person start with an outline and then fill in details systematically, or adopt a haphazard approach, slavishly copying detail after unrelated detail?

2. On object assembly tasks, do people use their knowledge of what the finished product should be to assist placement, or do they proceed in a trial and error fashion, attempting impossible or unreasonable juxtapositions?

3. Retention of spatial co-ordinates. Is the copy/drawing distorted in proportions; are features displaced, shifted to one side, rotated, altered in size, fragmented? Do they draw on top of the model instead of beside it? Are three-dimensional models reproduced as two-dimensional?

4. Can the person manage to draw angles and curves, intersect lines, maintain directionality, produce/inhibit closure?

5. Do they include all details, simplify the model or elaborate upon it?

6. Is there a tendency to concretisation, that is, abstract figures are copied as real objects they might resemble?

7. Do they make several attempts, touch up their effort, repeatedly drawing over lines already drawn?

8. Is there perseveration of strategies in completion, or in particular elements of designs?

Considerably more features than these have been used in marking constructional ability, but most of them (except the time taken, which some procedures measure) fall into the broad categories listed here. In general, these criteria discriminate between normal and brain-damaged populations (see works cited above) and are used within brain-damaged groups to separate (constructional) dyspraxics from non-dyspraxics.

Since it was established that CD may result from lesions of either hemisphere, attention has been focused on the above features for reasons other than simply distinguishing between dyspraxics and non-dyspraxics.

Clinicians and researchers have sought evidence from quantitative and qualitative performance to confirm whether left and right hemisphere CD represents two separate forms of dyspraxia.

Are There Two Constructional Dyxpraxias?

Quantitative Approaches

Earlier works (Piercy, Hécaen and De Ajuriaguerra, 1960; Benton and Fogel, 1962) maintained that CD due to right hemisphere lesions was both more frequent and more severe than CD due to left-sided lesions. While subsequent works (De Renzi and Faglioni, 1967; Black and Strub, 1976; Arena and Gainotti, 1978; Black and Bernard, 1984) have replicated this tendency, they have not always found the variation to be statistically significant.

One exception is the work of Mack and Levine (1981). They found a significantly greater deficit in connection with right retro-rolandic lesions over left-sided ones. However, it should be remembered that their test material (Figure 3.3) was designed with the intention of tapping right hemisphere visuo-perceptive skills rather than supposed executive skills of the left hemisphere. Also, Mack and Levine (1981, p. 528) themselves question whether or not their right brain-damaged group was truly representative.

The straightforward interpretation of the finding of more frequent and more severe CD after right-sided lesion is that processes underlying constructional ability have greater, or more crucial, representation in the right hemisphere. Several findings suggest, though, that the differences may be due to artifacts in selection and testing procedures.

For instance, the exclusion of (moderate to severe) dysphasics from left hemisphere groups because it was assumed they would not comprehend instructions, meant that some studies had severe cases only in their right lesioned population. Arena and Gainotti (1978) demonstrated that the quantitative differences in severity between right and left hemisphere CD were no longer significant when all dysphasics were retained in left hemispheric groups.

Another source of variation suspected of operating in unselected populations is the difference in severity related to the size and duration of lesion. Left posterior temporal and parietal lesions tend to be associated with dysphasia, while corresponding right-sided lesions are not. It is argued that language dysfunction is perceived by the sufferer as being more severe than the more subtle visual–spatial disorders accompanying right temporal–parietal lesions. Hence, in cases of neoplasm or degenerative changes, left-sided lesions are detected and help is sought before they are as severe as right-sided changes, which do not attract attention until later stages. After CVA's, without specific testing (cf. the woman described on p. 57), right cortical neuropsychological dysfunction is more likely to pass unnoticed or unappreciated for what it is, than more obvious dominant hemisphere disabilities. Arrigoni and De Renzi (1964) found significant quantitative differences between left and right CD patients. However, the differences between their scores became negligible when the two groups were matched for severity of lesion on a visual reaction time test.

One interpretation of the findings of De Renzi and Faglioni (1967) may explain why larger lesions are associated with right hemisphere CD. They postulated that constructional functions may be localised more discretely in the left and more diffusely in the right. Greater lesions would therefore be necessary to produce CD in right-sided brain damage. Black and Bernard (1984) found that lesion size made a comparatively minor contribution to the visual constructional deficits in their sample. Lesion size correlated significantly with CD scores only in the left retro-rolandic lesion group, and this they suspected might have been due to language rather than direct constructional factors.

The different commonly co-occurring disabilities between left- and right-sided lesions have also been suggested as skewing factors in severity ratings. Non-dominant hemisphere constructional dyspraxics have unilateral neglect and hemianopia more frequently than dominant hemisphere patients. Subjects are marked down for errors on some tests that may well result from hemi-inattention or visual field defects rather than from CD proper. Hence, quantitatively they appear more impaired, whereas in actual fact their poorer performance is not directly related to CD.

Certain studies (see below) rated severity according to independent judges' pronouncements on the qualitative integrity of drawings. As shown on pages 65 and 67, the type of qualitative errors made in right hemisphere CD are more likely to lead to the subjective impression of impairment than left-sided dyspraxics' errors (compare Figures 3.4 and 3.5).

Thus, it can be concluded that, as a group, right hemisphere CD patients score worse than left-sided ones. However, the importance of this for the understanding of CD is unclear, (a) because the differences have not always reached statistical significance, and (b) because these differences may be attributable to factors outside of the CD itself. For

Figure 3.4: Copy of Car, Using Right Hand, By a Man With a Left Parietal CVA

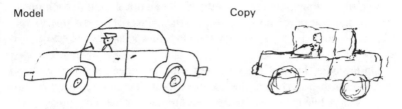

Model   Copy

Figure 3.5: Copy of Car, Using Right Hand by a Woman With a Right Frontoparietal CVA

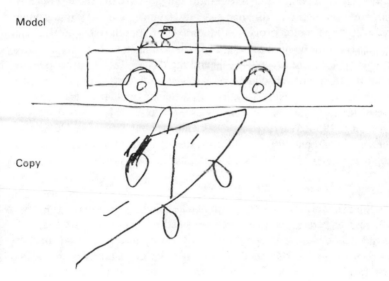

Model

Copy

this reason, others have sought to distinguish between right- and left-sided CD by other means, namely through qualitative error evaluation.

Qualitative Approaches

People who support a left–right qualitative distinction believe that CD in left- and right-sided lesions reflects a disruption to different underlying mechanisms. It has important consequences for rehabilitation if this is true.

Right hemisphere CD is seen as resulting from a disruption to visual–perceptual and visual–spatial processes. Thus, in right-sided CD the person may no longer retain the ability to view an object or task as a perceptual whole. Although individual parts of the stimuli may be recognised or manipulated correctly, their relationship with each other and the integration of all the parts to form a whole is lost due to the lack of a visual–perceptual model and loss of a visual check on the accuracy of attempts.

On the other hand, CD associated with left-sided lesions is viewed as a failure to programme the complex motor actions required to execute tasks, while the visual–spatial input remains intact. Obviously, such a simplified distinction is rather artificial since any constructional act demands input from both visual–spatial and motor planning for calculating plane, direction, co-ordination, speed and force of movements. The artificiality of separating these out ultimately leads to the same problems that are encountered, for instance, in trying to divide underlying phonology and motor processes in apraxia of speech (Chapter 4). The uniqueness of the ability lies precisely in the unification of the two strands.

This difficulty of completely separating the two factors probably explains the failure of subsequent research to confirm the initial optimism regarding the lateralising validity of particular qualitative error types. These characteristics have been reviewed in general by several writers (Duensing, 1953; Warrington, 1969; Gainotti and Tiacci, 1970; Hartje, Kerschensteiner and Sturm, 1975; De Renzi, 1982). Works dealing with the significance and validity of individual features are quoted below.

Alleged Right Hemisphere Features

The following errors have been claimed as being indicative of right-sided CD: loss of perspective; displacement and distortion of parts; loss of spatial relationship between parts; progressing in a piecemeal manner not relating one part to another. Duensing (1953) and Consoli (1979) view this loss of the perception of the whole at the expense of attention to detail by detail, as a main underlying factor in right-sided CD.

In right-sided CD, these errors and strategies lead to a fragmentation of the whole, giving it an 'exploded' appearance, and fragmentation may render the production unrecognisable, even to the person who constructed it.

Low critical evaluation, with poor recognition of errors, is also indicative of right-sided CD. Asked if the effort is satisfactory, even if it is, the person may say no, and proceed to make changes or add further features. Low critical evaluation may exist even in the presence of a model to copy and trace. Hécaen and Assal (1970) suggested that the presence of a model may even exacerbate the difficulty.

Figure 3.6: Copy of a House, Using Right Hand, By a Woman with a Right Frontoparietal CVA

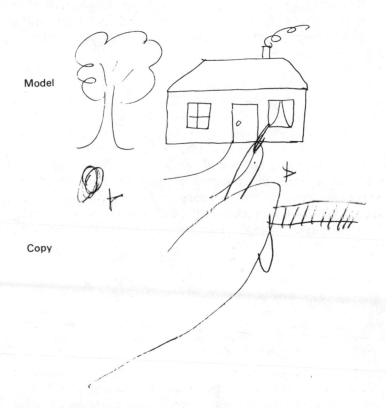

Model

Copy

Unwanted details are added in right-sided CD. These may be extra objects like the fence in Figure 3.6, or additional unrelated words or numbers. Copies tend to be rotated diagonally (see Figures 3.1b, 3.5, 3.6 and 3.7) with a predominance of lines sloping down to the bottom left (Piercy *et al.*, 1960). Crowding of copies to the right and neglect of features in the left (Figures 3.5 and 3.8) are also indicative. Gainotti, Miceli and Caltagirone (1977) rightly point out that these more likely originate from left-sided neglect than CD proper. Finally, execution is fluent and unhesitant, with bold, well-formed lines (Figure 3.9).

Alleged Left Hemisphere Features

The following errors have been claimed as being indicative of left-sided CD: poverty of detail, with copies being schematic or simplified (Figures

Figure 3.7: Drawing of a House, Without Model, By a Patient With a Right Frontoparietal CVA

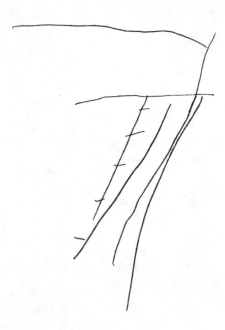

Figure 3.8: Drawing of a House, Without Model, By a Woman With a Right Frontoparietal CVA. This was drawn on a separate occasion to Figures 3.5, 3.6, 3.7 and 3.9

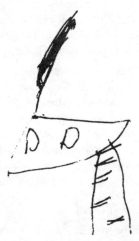

Figure 3.9: Drawing of House Following a Verbal Description (see text p. 75) By the Same Woman as in Figure 3.8

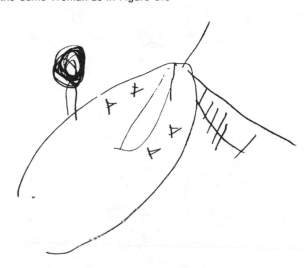

3.10, 3.11, 3.12); a cube might be reproduced as a square (Figure 3.13), for example, patient number three in Duensing's work (1953) produced a rough triangle when asked to draw a pear, and a loveheart was produced first as an 'M' and then on the fourth attempt as two juxtaposed parallelograms; Warrington *et al.* (1966) noted that acute angles tend to become right angles (for example, the points become blunter when a star is drawn (Figures 3.13, 3.14); angles may be reproduced as scrawls (Figures 3.13, 3.14 and 3.15), left open, or overlap ambiguously (Figures 3.10, 3.11); copies are reduced in size from the original (Figure 3.12) (see also Gainotti and Tiacci, 1970); there is a tendency to close in towards the model, overlap it or even to draw on top of it, both in paper and pencil and block tests (see Figures 3.10, 3.11 and 3.16); spatial relationships and overall recognisability are preserved, even though some features may be out of proportion; completion is slow, hesitant and laborious, with repeated false starts. The person may easily give up or even refuse to start in the first place because they feel they will fail. Figure 3.4 took almost five minutes to complete. Left hemisphere CD sufferers are heavily penalised on timed exercises. Mack and Levine (1981) take the slowness of left hemispherics as support for an underlying motor dysfunction.

Copying designs is done by slavishly drawing one detail after another. Thus, given sufficient time, left-sided CD sufferers may complete a task

Figure 3.10: Copy of House By a Man With a Left Temporoparietal CVA

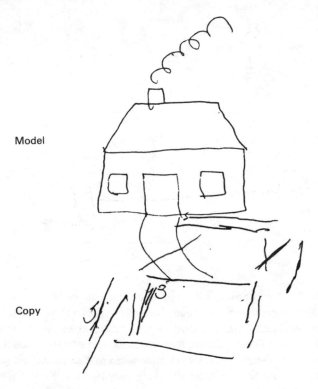

Model

Copy

satisfactorily. Their order of completion may be quite abnormal, however. Figure 3.4 represents a recognisable attempt at copying the model, but the sequence for drawing the parts was: bonnet and roof; steering wheel; driver; back window and boot; front bumper; door division; wheels; floor.

Finally, left-sided CD sufferers are aided by models and visual landmarks (dots, guidelines). This finding is supported by Hécaen and Assal (1970), though Duensing (1953) has stated that this is only true of less severe cases.

Are These Distinctions Valid and Reliable?

For each study that has claimed a particular feature to have lateralising value, there is another that has not. Warrington *et al.* (1966) submitted drawings of cubes and stars to a naïve judge, who failed to separate

Figure 3.11: Copy of Car By a Man With a Left Temporoparietal CVA

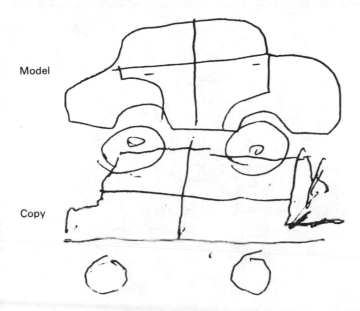

Model

Copy

them into left and right on the features of simplification and dislocation. He also failed to establish significant differences on the basis of relative size of the copy to the model, rotation, reiteration of lines already drawn and gaps or crossed lines instead of 'clean' angles.

Gainotti and Tiacci (1970), on tests of copying crosses and geometric designs, did not find the following features distinguished reliably between left and right hemisphere CD in their patients: (1) increased number of right angles; (2) alteration of relative size where there were several figures in one design; (3) increased size of the figures; (4) producing scrawls rather than recognisable attempts; (5) elements of perseveration; (6) closing in effect. All these characteristics had previously been alleged to separate right- and left-lesioned patients.

The distinguishing features that did reach statistical significance in Gainotti and Tiacci's (1970) study were, for left hemisphere CD: (1) reduced size of copy compared to the model; (2) loss of details, that is, simplification; (3) increased number of right angles on the copies of cubes and a rhombus; and (4) a tendency to reproduce angles as scrawls or curved lines.

For right hemisphere CD the significant features proved to be: (1) unilateral neglect; (2) piecemeal approach; (3) diagonal orientation of

Figure 3.12: Two Attempts At Copying a House By a Man With a Left Posterior Parietal CVA. He gave up on the first copy, realising it was wrong

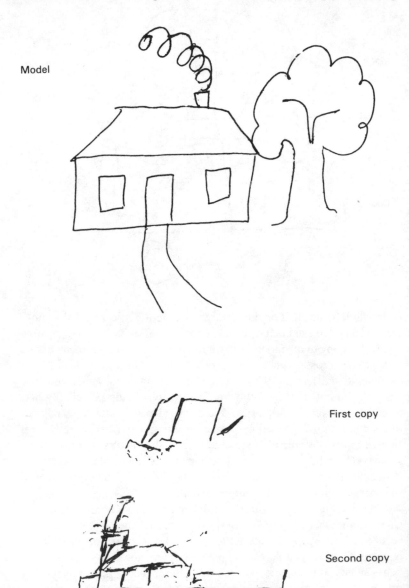

Model

First copy

Second copy

Figure 3.13: Copy of a Star and Cube. The same person produced Figures 3.4 and 3.14

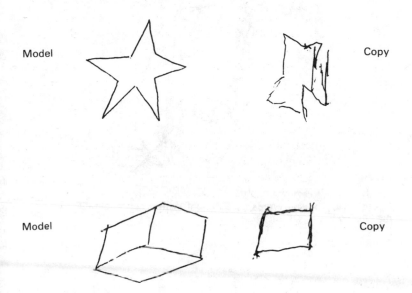

Model   Copy

Model   Copy

Figure 3.14: Drawing of a Five-pointed Star and Cube Without Models

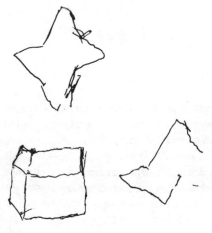

Figure 3.15: Free Drawing of a Car By the Same Person Who Drew Figures 3.12 and 3.16

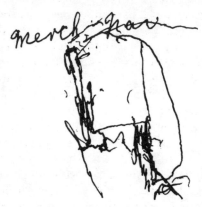

Figure 3.16: Copying Words By a Patient With a Left Parietal CVA. Note the closing in on 'sel' of 'chisel'

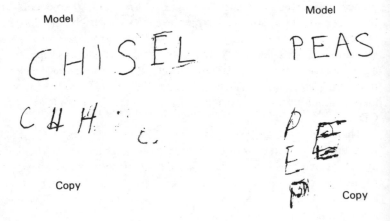

copies; (4) gross alterations in the spatial relations between figures if a design consisted of several figures; (5) tendency to overscore lines already drawn; and (6) inclusion of irrelevant script or material.

Gainotti *et al.* (1977) did not succeed in replicating the findings of Hécaen and Assal (1970) regarding the assistance given by landmarks. They found that if one compared the assistance given by landmarks only in the visual hemi-fields where no neglect or inattention would be expected, then no left–right difference emerged.

Deshayes, Cressard, Paulin *et al.* (1979) on the other hand did find that left-lesioned patients were helped by landmarks and that they tended to produce angles as curves, simplified diagrams and may produce unrecognisable drawings. They did not find slowness of execution, a typical left hemisphere trait. Their right hemisphere patients adopted a piecemeal approach, rotated copies diagonally and produced asymmetric drawings, in particular with left-sided neglect. They also added extra features. Deshayes *et al.* (1979) base their conclusions on clinical observation rather than statistical analysis.

As can be seen, the picture is far less clearcut than some texts would lead one to believe. This is illustrated by the figures in this chapter: Figures 3.6 to 3.9 were produced by a woman with a right frontoparietal infarct. Figure 3.7 is the result of the instruction 'draw a house'. Figure 3.9 is a free drawing, the patient having been told which features to include (that is, a description of the model subsequently given in Figure 3.6). Figure 3.6 is a direct copy; Figure 3.9 is a drawing from memory.

These drawings contain many of the features noted as typical of right hemisphere CD: incomplete left side; unrecognisability of drawings; exploded, fragmented drawings (in Figure 3.6 the cross-like details are the windows, the 'hook' underneath was supposed to be the door); a tendency to situate drawings diagonally (see Figure 3.5, by the same woman); and additional details (the railway track feature was supposedly a garden fence). However, to some extent, closing-in could be described in Figure 3.6; angles are either rounded or lines crossed over each other; there is simplification. Each of these features is typical of left hemisphere CD.

These figures should be compared with Figures 3.10 and 3.11, which were drawn by a man with a left temporoparietal lesion. Without the model for reference, Figure 3.10 would be unrecognisable. It shows additional material (the numbers); it could be described as fragmented; and it was completed without hesitation or slowness. These are features more usually linked with right hemisphere CD.

Similar conflict with supposed right–left distinctions can be seen in other figures. According to the criterion of 'recognisable or not', Figure 3.8 would have been drawn by a left hemisphere CD, and 3.15 by a right — and yet the reverse is true. By the same criterion Figures 3.7 and 3.8 would be seen as being drawn by a right and left hemisphere dyspraxic respectively, but they are both by the same right hemisphere patient. Figure 3.6 when compared to 3.7 suggests that the model aided construction, again contradicting claims that landmarks assist only left-lesioned patients. Figures 3.13 and 3.14 illustrate productions with and without a model by a left-hemisphere dyspraxic.

In answer to the question of whether or not there are characteristic errors or strategies that reliably differentiate right from left hemisphere CD, the answer must be no. At best, one can discern a general tendency. The more features present from one list, the more reliable the assignment of a left–right distinction. The uncertainty of relying on single criteria has been illustrated with examples from patients and the contrary views of experimental findings. Even those studies that have found in favour of certain features have been based only on a statistical tendency and not on absolute divisions. Gainotti and Tiacci (1970) provide a good example. In their study, errors found significantly greater in one hemisphere group were nevertheless found in the opposite group, too. Also, members of one group did not necessarily produce the errors established as more likely to occur in that group.

Underlying Mechanisms in Constructional Dyspraxia

Hand in hand with searches for hemispheric differences in qualitative performance, have gone attempts to prove that right and left hemisphere CD result from the breakdown of different underlying processes. A visual–spatial disorder has been postulated in right hemisphere patients and an executive motor dysfunction in left hemisphere patients.

Piercy and Smyth (1962) pointed out that if right hemisphere constructional dyspraxics suffer from a visual–spatial disorder, they alone should fail on visual–spatial perceptual tasks, while other dyspraxic and non-dyspraxic groups should not. Warrington and James (1967) reported a higher relationship between visual perceptual deficit and CD in right, but not left, hemisphere CD. Piercy and Smyth (1962) failed to uphold their hypothesis, though their study can be criticised for relying on Raven's progressive matrices as a measure for spatial perception. They are more a test of general intelligence. Arena and Gainotti (1978) found visual–perceptual deficits to be higher in their left brain-damaged group. They interpreted this as being due to the inclusion of dysphasics who had been excluded from other studies.

De Renzi (1982) has pointed out that one factor in producing the conflicting results is that the visual–perceptual assessments typically administered are only in general terms related to the visual–spatial demands of carrying out constructional tasks. These involve more the analysis of each line of a model with respect to its absolute orientation and articulation with neighbouring lines. The one study so far that has included line length and angle discrimination (Mack and Levine, 1981) did find a high correlation between constructional performance and visual–perceptual deficit in right but not left hemisphere subjects.

Attempts to prove an executive neurodynamic pathology in left hemisphere CD have been directed chiefly to examining the effects on performance of factors that it was considered should assist motor control. Warrington *et al.* (1966) encouraged patients to copy figures of simple outline (unstructured) and ones with internal details (structured). They predicted that simple outlines should be easier for left hemispheric patients, whereas structured figures (where the internal markings should aid definition of the spatial relationships) should be easier for right-sided cases. Their hypothesis was not borne out. The contrasting findings regarding the effects of landmarks, which should help motor planning, have been mentioned above.

Consoli (1979) observed different strategies in right and left hemisphere dyspraxics in the execution of the template matching task (Figure 3.2). In summary, normal constructional praxis was seen by Consoli as comprising, among other things, three essential and inseparable components: reception and analysis of visual–spatial data; logical comparison operations; and the establishment of a gestural motor programme. The role of the right hemisphere was interpreted as having a synthetic, global spatial role, and the left a sequential, analytic role. In right-sided lesions, therefore, the left hemisphere is able to carry out a sequential analysis of the material to be copied and constructed, but the global recognition and organisation of the information is impaired. In left-sided lesions, the global form is maintained because of the intact right hemisphere, but the transfer of the visual detail to an effective motor plan is short-circuited — giving a slow performance, without a logical motor plan, though, given sufficient time, the person can compensate for this through slavish attention to each visually processed detail. Semenza, Denes, D'Urso *et al.* (1978) found left-lesioned patients less able than normal people and right-lesioned patients to use a global strategy in copying simple drawings, as opposed to a piece by piece approach.

The question has arisen whether CD is a visual–perceptual disorder in both left and right hemisphere cases with motor dysfunction stemming from the presence of other dyspraxias.

Ideomotor dyspraxia is not a constant finding in left sided CD. De Ajuriaguerra *et al.* (1960a) found that 39.8 per cent of their left-lesion population had CD, but only 18.9 per cent of them had ideomotor dyspraxia. Of the 47 individuals with ideomotor dyspraxia, only 34 also showed CD. Duensing (1953) distinguished between classical ideational dyspraxia and ideational configurational disturbance (his term for so-called executive CD), but conceded that the distinction was far from remarkable. Essentially, he interpreted classical ideational dyspraxia as a disruption of frequently practised, largely automatic actions reproduced in everyday life, while in CD the production of new actions is disturbed.

Signoret and North (1979) see ideational and left-sided constructional dyspraxia as one and the same. Others (De Ajuriaguerra and Tissot, 1969) have drawn a distinction between ideational dyspraxia as relating to concrete action space, while CD relates to Euclidean space.

Le Doux (1979) has put forward another view based on evidence from split-brain patients. He noted that the (right-hemisphere controlled) left hand performs more or less normally on constructive tasks, but that the right hand does not. This suggests that the left hemisphere has minimal spatioconstructive ability. But why, then, do left-hemisphere lesions cause CD? Le Doux proposed that constructional praxis processes are sited wholly in the right parietal-occipital lobes. A left posterior lesion causes CD because it disconnects the motor areas for the right hand from the right parieto-occipital region. According to Le Doux, a right-sided lesion will cause bilateral CD, while a left-sided lesion will bring about a unilateral right CD. This view awaits experimental confirmation, although readers are referred to Brown, Leader and Blum (1983) and Leischner (1983).

The problems of isolating any one function in the genesis of CD may be rooted in the fact that, as with so many higher cortical functions, construction is not simply a consecutive or simultaneous addition of several independent processes, but a result of the concerted interaction between them. Visual–spatial perception may be associated predominantly with the right hemisphere, but for praxic purposes the necessary spatial information is not a pre-packaged whole simply to be run off parallel to the motor act. The visual–spatial planning needs to be mapped on to the motor programme, which, in turn, takes place in time and in space. Therefore, it requires constant spatial reference and adjustment. One is presented with a situation similar to that outlined for apraxia of speech (Chapter 4). Articulation is taken not simply as the underlying syntax and phonology plus a motor component. The two facets are seen to influence each other in a much more complex manner.

As with the question of left–right qualitative variation in errors, the problem of differing underlying mechanisms in left and right CD remains unsolved. It still has to be clarified whether visual–spatial representation is uni- or bilateral. If it is bilateral, what is the nature of the representation in each hemisphere? Is the right hemisphere capable of motor control independent of the left hemisphere? Split brain studies suggest that it is. What strategies can be used to circumvent the difficulty faced in trying to separate out for experimental purposes visual–spatial and motor processes? Studies to date have required elements of both, even though the possible influence of one has been taken as minimal.

Answers to these and associated questions have clinical as well as experimental significance. If it is true that left-sided lesions produce only a unilateral CD, the intactness of the left hand could be exploited in rehabilitation. If there is a left–right motor–visual–spatial divide, then therapeutic intervention would need to be directed at the relevant underlying breakdown. If it is a question of different types of visual–spatial processing or visuo-motor functioning being impaired in either hemisphere, intervention would only be directed efficiently if it were designed to remediate the true disruption.

Associated Disorders

Occasionally, CD may be an isolated finding, but more often than not it is only one of several dysfunctions. The clinician's task will usually be not just to establish the presence of CD, but also to gauge how far the person's difficulties stem from the CD and how far from the co-occurring disorders.

Fortunately, for clinicians, the disabilities associated with left and right hemisphere lesions can be described with more certainty than the nature of errors or underlying mechanisms of CD.

Right Hemisphere Disorders

Assuming that primary receptive (visual, haptic, auditory) functions are normal, and having excluded or taken into account visual field defects, the main disorders associated with right hemisphere CD concern the perception and interpretation of the visual–spatial world.

Visual Agnosia. This is rare in its pure form, but elements of it may interfere with constructional tasks. In extreme cases, the person cannot name on sight objects or pictures. In less severe cases, they might describe features of the object. On the basis of inferences from certain features, the person may misname, misuse or miscopy the object. An apple might be called a ball, a tooth-brush a screwdriver. For its part, this behaviour must be distinguished from optic dysphasia (p. 36; Larrabee *et al.*, 1985), where the patient is unable to name objects presented visually, yet can show that he recognises the objects, either by gesturing their use, matching them to a picture, pointing to them when they are named, or naming them correctly to tactile or auditory stimulus.

In the absence of auditory or haptic defects, the visual dysgnosic may be assisted in recognising an object if they hear the sound commonly linked with it (telephone, saw), or if they can feel it. Placing the object in its familiar context may also help. In a personal case, a patient, when shown her own clock out of context said it was 'some kind of round thing'. Later, she labelled it correctly when asked what it was before it had been removed from its usual bedside place.

Simultanagnosia. Another form of defective recognition is when the person may be able to label individual features but not combine the knowledge to analyse a whole object, picture or word. On looking at a picture of someone lighting a cigarette, the patient may simply describe it or draw it as a cigarette, without even mentioning the smoker or the match. Examining a comb, the patient may observe that 'these are spikes', but not relate them to their function or part in the whole. This behaviour has been variously termed, with different shades of meaning, 'amorphosynthesis', 'simultanagnosia' and 'disorder of simultaneous form perception'. Simultanagnosia is used here to label the behaviour described without any intention of supporting a particular theoretical explanation. Some see this as the basis of the piecemeal approach and loss of spatial relationships in CD. For further discussion, readers are referred to Hécaen and Albert (1978) and Heilman and Rothi (1985).

Sensory Extinction. Visual extinction may impair constructional praxis if the person is unable to monitor the movements of both hands simultaneously, or if he is incapable of attending at the same time to his hand and pencil, and the paper and drawing. This difficulty has also been implicated in optic ataxia (p. 44).

Sensory extinction has been pointed to as a cause of disability in estimating angles, depth of field, relative distance and perception of movement, all of which have clear consequences for praxis.

Hemi-inattention. This may relate to visual, tactile and/or auditory stimuli. Neglect of, or inattention to, objects or parts of objects will correspondingly impair perception and interpretation of objects, pictures or situations. Inattention and neglect may be manifested in graphic representations of objects, faces and bodies, both from models and from memory (Figures 3.5 and 3.9). The reinterpretation of space required to make sense of the world with one half missing may also mean that even the intact half is perceived quite differently from normal.

Topographical Disorders. This area comprises a number of distinct problems that cannot be covered in detail here. People may be unable to orientate themselves spatially, even in familiar surroundings. They cannot find their way to the shops, around the house or back to their bed on the ward. They may be unable to point out well-known landmarks on a map of their own locality, and cannot trace on it the route they take to work or to the shops. This may extend to an inability to describe the routes verbally. Inserting the names of familiar cities, countries or seas on a map may prove difficult or impossible. Topographical disorders proper are to be distinguished from disorientation due to inattention, neglect or dementia.

Spatial Dyslexia and Dysgraphia. A consequence of visual spatial disorders may be characteristic reading and writing difficulties (see Hécaen and Albert, 1978; Benson, 1979). Words may be missed in sentences, and lines may be missed out or repeated. Errors related to spatial imperception occur: 'saw' may be read as 'was' or 'aws', 'gape' for 'page'. Visually similar letters or words may be confused: 'ship' for 'shop', w for m, or b for d.

Where unilateral neglect is present, text in the neglected half may be omitted. Long words, in particular, may be misread: 'railway station' may be read as 'station', 'carrot' as 'rot', '721' as '21'. If the resultant error word does not fit the context and the person is aware of the mismatch, a more apt reading may be substituted: for example, 'dripping' (water tap) was read as 'spring' by one patient. This is an example in reading of the wider reinterpretation of the environment that may take place in hemianopic/hemineglect patients.

Spatial dyslexia is often accompanied by a spatial dysgraphia and dyscalculia. In writing, the syntax of sentences, the morphology of words and spelling are intact, essentially. This underlines the fact that it is not a language-based disorder. However, resulting from the commonly co-occurring hemispatial neglect, the writing tends to occupy the right-hand side of the page only, with a tendency for the left-hand margin to increase as the writer proceeds down the page. Even when ruled lines are present as guides, or even in tracing exercises in severe cases, the text may tend to spread diagonally instead of horizontally across the page, or the line may undulate or take a staircase form. The letters may also show a diagonal slant untypical for the writer. The spatial relationships

Figure 3.17: Writing by (a) Patient With a Left Temporoparietal Infarct Using the Preferred Right Hand, and (b) Letters to Dictation By a Patient With a Left Frontal Subarachnoid Haemorrhage Using the Left Non-preferred Hand

(a)

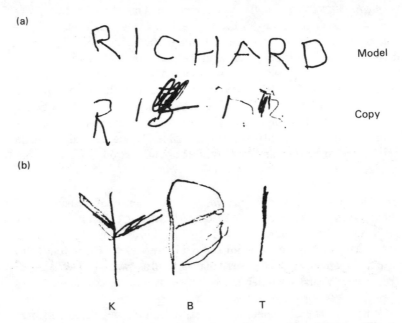

Model

Copy

(b)

K   B   T

between words may be lost due to irregular spacing of letters (Figure 3.18). The graphemes themselves are generally well formed, though there may be instances of extra strokes — especially letters such as u, w, m, n and l (Figure 3.19). Compare this to the characteristics of dyspraxic dysgraphia (Figures 3.16 and 3.17).

Left Hemisphere Disorders

The main associated disorders here are language- and praxis-related. Primary sensory and motor dysfunctions may be present, as might visual field defects.

Language. It is important, as always, to ensure that a person is not said to have CD simply because they misunderstood the verbal instructions. Vigilance is especially required with suspected CD since it is likely to co-occur with those dysphasias where comprehension, both spoken and written, is worst. Even conduction dysphasics (page 106), who appear to have relatively good understanding, may miss the subtleties of precise instructions

Figure 3.18: Writing to Dictation With Her Right Hand, by a Woman With a Right Parietal-occipital CVA

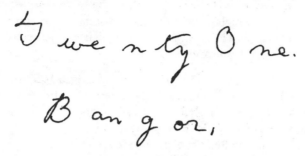

Figure 3.19: James McLaughlin By a Patient With a Right Cerebral Closed Head Injury

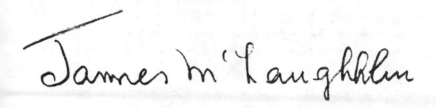

Reading and writing problems are liable to be language-based in left brain damage. However, dyspraxic dysgraphia may be found.

Dyspraxic Dysgraphia. Cases of dyspraxic dysgraphia after left hemisphere lesion without any language involvement have been reported (see Hécaen and Albert, 1978; Benson, 1979; Margolin, 1984; Roeltgen, 1985, for reviews). However, it usually co-occurs with dysphasic dysgraphia, or the syndrome of agraphia with alexia, where spoken language is relatively preserved apart from possible naming difficulties.

Patients have difficulty forming graphemes both spontaneously and to dictation. Letters are reversed, inverted, distorted, incomplete or produced as scrawls. Copying may also be impaired, or performed with much effort, but without necessarily understanding what has been written (Figures 3.16, 3.17). Additionally, holding and manipulating the pencil may be affected. Using cut-out letters or typewriters may or may not help according to the degree of accompanying language disruption.

Other Dyspraxias. CD may co-occur with ideational and/or ideomotor dyspraxia. The exact distinction between ideational and constructional dyspraxia is disputed (page 78).

Hemi-inattention. Right-sided neglect or inattention sometimes results from left hemisphere lesions, but not as regularly as left-sided neglect occurs after right hemisphere injury.

Gerstmann's Syndrome. CD is frequently mentioned as a fifth element to the tetrad of symptoms of alleged Gerstmann's syndrome — the other four being finger agnosia, right–left disorientation, dyscalculia and pure agraphia. The validity of the concept of Gerstmann's syndrome has been questioned (compare Benton, 1961; Poeck and Orgass, 1966; Roeltgen, Sevush and Heilman, 1983). The independent status of finger agnosia and right–left disorientation have also been debated (p. 132). It is not possible to debate these issues in detail. The point is to draw to clinicians' notice the possible co-appearance of CD and apparent right–left disorientation, finger agnosia, dyscalculia and dysgraphia. The view held here is that all these features will require further differential diagnosis. They may derive from language, visual–spatial, attentional or praxic difficulties.

Certain disorders may be present after lesions of either hemisphere. Ocular motor disorders (Chapter 5) may affect scanning of objects and pictures (Yarbus, 1967; Tyler, 1969), which may in turn determine the quality of patients' constructional skills. Motor impersistence (p. 43) may influence performance, as also may optic ataxia and the other disorders outlined in Chapter 2 as clouding the picture in other dyspraxias.

More anterior lesions are liable to involve more prominent primary motor and sensory deficits, while more posterior lesions may be accompanied, too, by occipital lobe dysfunctions, which have not been discussed here.

On occasions, a differential diagnosis will be necessary between CD as a result of localised damage or as part of a picture of dementia. Clearly, dyspraxia assessment alone will not decide the answer, but analysis of dyspraxic errors, and language and other assessments and case history details may help. One would search in such instances, first, for signs of whether praxic, linguistic and other disorders fall into relatively well-defined clinical categories — CD, ideational, ideomotor dyspraxia, and so on; sensory/Wernicke's or anomic dysphasia, or alexia with agraphia, and so on; primary motor and sensory deficits; and modality specific 'memory' disorders, or definable amnestic syndromes. Then one has to consider whether the pictures of disruption in the separate areas are explainable on the basis of a single lesion site, dysfunction of a particular process, or whether they represent consequences of disruption to multiple or diffuse areas of brain. A personal case demonstrates this problem.

Case Report. A previously healthy, determinedly independent, 71-year-old widower was admitted to a general medical ward having been found in the local supermarket trying to get into a cupboard and talking 'nonsense'. Hospital staff did not attempt to take a case history from him on admission because of his jargon language. His family reported memory difficulties over the previous months. He had become neglectful of household chores, leaving pots unwashed and jars and packets not put away. He had stopped changing his clothes regularly and looked generally scruffy. Bills had been left unpaid. A lightswitch he had started to repair (he was a former electrician) had been left with bare wires hanging out of the wall. A relative who lived far away had rung up to see what was wrong, having not received his regular letter. He was further described as having become dithery and clumsy, bumping into things and dropping things, all of which was quite out of character.

Medical examination showed no cranial nerve involvement, no primary motor or sensory impairment, and no other systemic or local abnormalities. The only suggestion of an abnormal finding was an equivocal reaction to menace from the right.

On the ward he was agitated, depressed and frequently spoke jargon, predominantly English. He knew where he lived, who he was, and that he was now in hospital, though he could not always supply the names. Neither could he write down the names. He was disoriented in his immediate surroundings, and had difficulty finding his way to the toilet and back to his bed.

Language assessment established that he had a mild comprehension loss for spoken input and moderate–severe loss for written information. A marked anomia was present in expressive language. On naming objects, pictures or persons, there was either zero response, for which he apologised, or semantic paraphasic errors. The essential observation was that the paraphasic substitutions were within category and clearly related to the target word. Discourse analysis showed no disruption, and while his conversation was peppered with paraphasic errors and circumlocutions, overall there was coherence, relevance to the topic and awareness of difficulties on the listener's part. He was acutely aware of his errors.

Written expression was impossible. He was unable to form letters, and could only copy capital letters with great difficulty (Figures 3.12, 3.15 and 3.16 are his). The family confirmed that the way in which he was speaking was what they had termed 'nonsense'. He himself said he had not written to his relative because he could no longer work out how to write. Not knowing what had happened to himself, he had not wanted to admit this to his family. For the same reason, the bills had not been paid. An additional problem was that he was unable to check if they were right.

Visual–praxic assessment similarly demonstrated specific disabilities. There was a degree of right neglect, mainly for extracorporeal space. On body part identification, as well as difficulties locating some parts, there was also confusion between whether to point to his own or the examiner's body. Although he had difficulties finding his way to the toilet and back to his bed, he could locate himself by reasoning where he must be on the basis of the direction he had come from, where he had last been, and from known landmarks in the ward. This demonstrated that the disorientation was more likely founded on the hemi-neglect and in-attention rather than real loss of topographical memory, reasoning or general confusion. He stated that on the day of admission he had been wanting to get out of the supermarket and thought the door he was trying was the exit.

There was no apparent ideomotor dyspraxia and sequencing of several simple movements was intact, for example, pouring a cup of tea and adding sugar and milk. However, there was severe impairment on more complex sequences and actions. A dressing dyspraxia was present, with errors both of orientation of garments and order of putting on. Asked to fit a new fuse in a plug and reassemble it, he found the task impossible, despite being able to verbalise where things should go. There was a marked disability on graphic tasks (see Figure 3.16; note the marked closing-in of 'SEL' in 'chisel'). On copying, he demonstrated reduction in size, simplification and hesitant, effortful execution. He was well aware of these difficulties.

He himself reported that he had become untidy at home partly because he could not always find straightaway where things should be placed, although he knew where they ought to be, and partly because, even if he did find the drawer or cupboard, he could not always organise things properly inside them.

Aside from the dressing dyspraxia, the dirty washing had another plausible explanation. He had once been burgled and so kept his wardrobe and chest of drawers (where he kept his valuables as well as his clean clothes) locked with a lock and padlock. He had great difficulty manipulating his keys to find the correct one, insert it into the lock and then dismantle the padlock, as well as reversing the process. Because he only sometimes succeeded at this, he was only able to change into clean clothes on those occasions. The neglected lightswitch was also explicable on the basis of CD. He related how he had been able to unscrew the parts relatively easily, but found it impossible to reassemble.

The forgetfulness and memory problem that the family initially reported referred partly to the lightswitch and jars lying around. They felt he had forgotten to attend to them, whereas from assessment and his own history, it was apparent that he had not forgotten about them. Rather, he was well aware of his negligence, and his difficulties in completing the tasks could be traced to specific deficits — CD and visual spatial disorientation.

The other memory problems claimed by the family related to his semantic paraphasic errors. They felt he had 'forgotten' their names and what various everyday objects were called. On memory testing, he showed no deficit in recall for distant or recent events in his own life or world history. He was able to order them chronologically and contextually. Immediate recall on verbal memory lay within normal limits making allowance for his dysphasia.

Functionally, a diagnosis of circumscribed lesion was indicated on the basis of behaviours that could be accounted for by well-defined and recognisable dysfunctions. The isolated dysfunctions could all be linked with a lesion in a specific area, as opposed to several non-associated areas or diffuse damage. In this case, the man presented a relatively clear-cut example of angular gyrus syndrome (Benson, Cummings and Tsai, 1982).

It was concluded that he had suffered a minor CVA or series of transient ischaemic attacks several months previously. Although the man and his family had noticed the behavioural consequences of this, they had not appreciated what might have been underlying the symptoms. This had led to the false impression of a progressive onset. Close questioning revealed that the onset of symptoms could be placed fairly definitely in time. He had suffered an extension of the stroke on the morning of admission.

Localisation of Lesions Causing Constructional Dyspraxia

Classically, CD has been linked with parietal, in particular lower posterior parietal, damage (Hyvärinen, 1982; Marinkovic, Kovacevic and Kostic, 1984). Statistical reviews (De Ajuriaguerra *et al.*, 1960; Black and Strub, 1976) have shown this link to be of a relative rather than absolute nature.

CD was found by them in purely temporal and occipital lesions, as well as combinations of these with parietal lesions and parietal lesions alone. CD is not infrequently found with frontal involvement (De Ajuriaguerra *et al.*, 1960a; Black and Strub, 1976; Truelle, Fardoun, Delestre *et al.*, 1979). This is not surprising considering the planning and controlling role assumed in the frontal lobes, a point emphasised by Luria and Tsvetkova (1964).

It has also been described in association with subcortical damage. Brown (1972) reported it in subcortical dementia (progressive supra-nuclear palsy). Agostoni *et al.* (1983) found CD after basal ganglia and thalamic infarcts. Villardita, Smirni, Le Pira *et al.* (1982) found visuo–spatial and CD disturbances in Parkinsonian patients, independent of mental deterioration. Where the latter was present, it only served to heighten the disability. They surmised that reduced ocular motor skills may have had a contributory effect, but also pointed to the profusion of basal ganglia–frontal cortex interconnections and the implications of this for planning. Boller, Passafiume, Keefe *et al.* (1984) confirmed visuo–spatial impairment in Parkinson's disease as a feature independent of other elements of the disorder.

Cambier *et al.* (1980) established CD, hemi-neglect and other features of parietal damage as a result of right thalamic infarct. Cambier *et al.* (1983) described patients with infarcts of the anterior choroidal artery which compromised the thalamo-cortical (retro-rolandic) fibres passing through the posterior arm and retrolenticular segment of the internal capsule. According to the side of the lesion, the neuropsychological picture was either of right or left parietal-type symptoms. CD also results from callosal lesions, as discussed on pages 131 to 132.

CD is a sequela of all the usual causes of brain damage. It has also been reported by Worrall and Gillham (1983) as a slowly developing sequela of administration of lithium within the normal therapeutic range. The impairment, which included also mild dysphasia and subjective memory difficulties, resolved after suspension of the lithium regime.

Conclusion

A disorder of visuo-motor co-ordination has been described in which the ability of the person to manipulate objects in space is impaired. The errors that distinguish constructional dyspraxics from other dyspraxics and normal people are relatively clear. However, determining whether sub-groups of errors exist corresponding to different hemispheric involvement or separate underlying dysfunctions remains undecided. Other disabilities with which CD commonly co-occurs have been mentioned, emphasising that assessment and rehabilitation of CD require not only attention to praxic elements, but a broader view of the context in which it occurs.

4   APRAXIA OF SPEECH

Although apraxia of speech was the first of the dyspraxias to be described explicitly, it is also the one around which most controversy has raged. To attempt a detailed definition would be to cross a swamp that has minefields on the islands. The central feature is a difficulty with the voluntary production of the sounds that go to make up spoken language, despite adequate muscle power and range of movements. In trying to say 'Put the TV on the table', someone suffering from apraxia of speech might say what sounds like 'A 'pud the 'chee 'B nond 'tail'ble' (' indicates a stressed syllable). There will be distortions of a sound on one occasion but not another (t in chee and tailble), anticipation of sounds (non, tailble), and apparent addition (apud), substitution (b for v), and omission of sounds (not instanced here). However, such a straightforward view hides over a century of heated debate, which has spawned a catalogue of definitions and labels that are signposts to the history of neurological and linguistic thinking over that time (see reviews by Darley, Aronson and Brown, 1975; Messerli, 1983).

Apraxia of speech (AS) has been termed aphemia, Broca's aphasia, baby Broca's (Mohr, Pessin, Finkelstein *et al.*, 1978; Mohr, 1980), anarthria (Lebrun, 1982; Messerli, 1983), efferent motor aphasia (Luria, 1973), peripheral motor dysphasia, sensorimotor impairment, syndrome of phonetic disintegration, and countless more.

Issues involved have centred round whether AS is a language disorder, and therefore a type of dysphasia, or whether it is a motor disorder, independent of any linguistic considerations and therefore a dyspraxia. Obviously, if the question was that clear cut, one would have expected some reasonable answers by now. Alas, the initial question merely raises a host of further problems. If it is a language disorder, which part of the language system is involved? What role does semantic, syntactic and morphological impairment play in the picture? Is it a disruption only to the sound system (phonology)? If so, is it at a high conceptual level of planning, or some lower level?

If it is a motor disorder, does it relate only to speech sound production? Is there a direct link between it and oral dyspraxia? Is it a disorder of retrieval, initiation, sequencing or of transition from one segment to the next?

Alternatively, can one ever separate out the several contributing processes to speech production? If not, and the disorder lies in the nature of the relationship between the linguistic and motor components, where precisely does the breakdown occur? At what stage in planning are the abstract sound strings and motor programmes mapped on to each other? Are sounds or words stored with some kind of motor representation? How do the sound and motor systems cope with the varying spatio-temporal contexts in which sounds occur?

It is impossible to deal with all these issues in one chapter. More detailed reviews can be found in Buckingham (1979); Kelso and Tuller (1981); Rosenbek, Kent and La Pointe (1984) and Roy and Square (1985).

These questions echo many of the problems posed in the understanding of other dyspraxias. For example, the dividing line between ideational, ideomotor and limb–kinetic dyspraxia, or the arguments over the nature of ideational dyspraxia. They are close to the issues in constructional dyspraxia in trying to separate out visual–spatial perceptual elements from motor aspects in planning. In constructional dyspraxia the difficulty lies at the confluence between a conceptual, abstract planning process and the specific action requirements (which themselves must derive from an abstract planning level) for the realisation of the concept.

At the interface, the dysfunction can be seen to lie not in either of the components separately, but precisely in their interaction. Hence it is no surprise that such a disorder as AS should manifest elements of dysfunction from the linguistic and the more purely motor bases. The view implicit in this chapter is that an understanding of AS will come from an appreciation of the duality of the speech production process.

The underlying difficulty is not for programming just any volitional oral movements, but for movements specific to the externalisation of the linguistic sound system. Given this view, it is no surprise that word class, word frequency, position of words in utterances and syntactic complexity, all strictly speaking non-phonological and non-motor factors, nevertheless influence the likelihood of motor accuracy (see Whitaker, 1983; Rosenbek *et al.*, 1984). Likewise, errors could be expected that are describable (some would say accountable for, see p. 96) as disordered phonological processes. Alongside these one should also expect distortions of segments and transitions between segments and distortions over whole utterances that are better understood as motor dysfunction (see p. 98).

The bias of this book is a clinical one, and so it is not intended to delve here deeply into theoretical considerations. Relevant preferences are given when contentious areas are passed. The theoretical side is more than of academic interest, though, since ultimately proper rehabilitative measures can only be devised when these issues are resolved.

What does the disorder around which all the controversy centres sound like? The following gives a brief picture, before going on to introduce treatment areas.

Clinical Presentation

Functional characteristics naturally vary with severity. They also vary with the prominence of associated features. So-called apraxia of speech rarely occurs as an isolated phenomenon. Some have been reported in the literature (Seinsch, 1981; Square, Darley and Sommers, 1982) but normally there is an accompanying dysphasia, as well as co-existing motor defects — hemiparesis, ideomotor, limb-kinetic and oral dyspraxia.

The sufferer may appear mute in severe cases. Attempts at vocalisation produce at most non-specific non-verbal movement, but no phonation. The person may just open their mouth, move their tongue, thrust the head forwards and expire forcefully, but be unable to make any sound. Despite this, they may give normal phonation when coughing, sneezing or yawning, or 'out of the blue' when trying to attract someone's attention. Typically, they are unable to repeat the call they have just made if asked.

David and Bone (1984) described a patient where the apraxia seemed to be restricted to laryngeal function. Hartman (1984) has discussed the differentiation of neurogenic laryngeal dysfunctions, including those found in AS.

In less severe cases, or previously severe cases later in the recovery process, the person may be able to utter vocalic sounds, but inconsistently, and not specific sounds to imitation. A person with severe dyspraxia is likely to display more attempts at vocalisation than the individual with overall severe dysphasia, and these attempts are usually accompanied by much gestural behaviour and signs of frustration.

The above assumes that the patient is co-operative and that their comprehension and orientation to the task are adequate (see sections headed Assessment and Differential Diagnosis).

In less severe impairment, the amount of vocalisation increases, with consonantal sounds appearing alongside the attempts at vocalic productions. Isolated words may appear sporadically. This not only adds to the sufferer's frustration of the sufferer, but may also add to his depression. They hear themselves utter a word and then, after fruitless attempts to reproduce it, will realise that it was only a fleeting success. One feature of AS is that it is as much a surprise to the speaker as to the listener when these words arise out of the blue. This behaviour may be interpreted as negative, lazy or obstinate if the true nature of AS has not been explained and if people do not appreciate why their relative, friend or patient might be able to say a word on one occasion, but not again. The impression of negativeness may be reinforced because, frequently, the words that appear are curses, even if the person was not known previously as one to use bad language.

Other words, or even phrases, that may be relatively (not necessarily absolutely) easy to produce are social exchanges (so-called reflexive speech) and 'automatic' sequences. Thus, as someone enters the room and bids 'Good-morning' the person with AS may reply 'Good-morning' perfectly clearly, and yet later on be unable to repeat it in an apparently simple repetition exercise. The same applies to 'Please', 'Thank you', 'Yes', 'No', 'Hello', 'Goodbye', 'Stop', and so on, in 'live' situations.

Likewise, the patient may be heard to utter clearly asides such as 'I can't say that' or 'Oh, my goodness, this is terrible'. The person with less severe AS can also usually produce overlearned series, such as counting or the days of the week, better than spontaneous speech, especially if cued in to start. Similarly, proverbs or the second half of common pairs (knife and . . ., salt and . . .) may be ably completed if someone says the first part for them, despite the person being unable to name fork or pepper in isolation.

Songs, prayers and poems earlier learned by heart may be elicited in appropriate situations, though the person is unable to say isolated lines or words from them. These features are also true of many dysphasics, so the occurrence of such behaviour should not be taken as pathognomic of AS.

In milder cases where conversation is possible, speech is usually described as non-fluent. The flow of talk is slow, and there are abnormal pauses between words or even within words. The pauses are observed to be filled with silent groping and struggle to gain articulatory postures. These efforts are frequently in vain and pronunciations may be off-target. An essential feature is that they are seldom far off-target and the intended word is usually apparent through the distortion. The person may make attempts at self-correction as they are well aware of the errors.

Another hallmark often claimed of AS is that individual sounds or words are not invariably mispronounced. The same sound or word with which the person showed difficulty on one occasion may be clearly spoken a few sentences later.

The overall slowed rate of speaking, the interruptions by the silent posturing and the tendency to even stress and even spacing of syllables results in an altered pattern of intonation. This may give the impression that the person is speaking in a strange dialect, or that they are foreign, particularly in mild cases. Indeed, one of the areas of differential diagnosis of AS may be with the so-called 'foreign accent syndrome' (Whitaker, 1983).

The patient of Monrad-Krohn (1947), after her initial dysphasia had resolved, sounded like a French or German person, despite having had no contact whatsoever with these languages. Patient Sm.-Sok. of Luria (1948, translated 1963) and the woman patient of Square and Mlcoch (1983) provide further examples.

All of these difficulties with pronunciation are disproportionate to what one might expect from the degree and locus of any decrease in muscle tone, power or co-ordination. They are also out of phase with what one would expect on the basis of their relatively spared language comprehension. They may be independent of the degree of any co-occurring oral, non-verbal dyspraxia.

Figure 4.1: Words Written By a Woman Suffering From a Relatively Pure Case of Apraxia of Speech

In purer cases of AS, writing is relatively spared (see Figure 4.1, written by a woman unable at the time to produce even single-word, intelligible utterances), though usually, owing to the presence of dysphasia, comparing spoken and written production will not necessarily assist in diagnosis or management.

Pronunciation Characteristics of Apraxia of Speech

Error Types

Pronunciation is intended here as a neutral descriptive term instead of the more contentious labels such as articulation, phonetic, phonological or linguistic. As already stated, AS sufferers mispronounce words, but how and why?

Analyses of errors (Deal and Darley, 1972; Trost and Canter, 1974; Dunlop and Marquardt, 1977) suggest that the likelihood of derailment of an articulatory gesture increases with the complexity of motor setting of the vocal tract (air stream, vocal cords, pharynx, soft palate, tongue, lips, mandible) required for its production, or transition from one setting to the next. It should be noted that it is the articulatory movement that is derailed, not the listener's or speaker's auditory target. The sound heard in the listener's ear is only the product of the articulatory activity. Such confusion between production and perception and between psychological and physical phenomena have been responsible for much earlier controversy over AS.

The implications of the articulatory complexity observation mean that affricates (ch in chair, j in jar) are expected to be more susceptible to error than fricatives (sh in shop, v and c in vice), which in turn are more difficult than plosives (p, t, k, b, d, g, as in pet, dog, kid). Plosives tend to be more difficult than laterals (l in loud), followed by nasals (m, n, ng), with vowels being the easiest of all. This is group data and variance at individual level is found.

By the same token, clusters of sounds, especially consonantal, requiring complex settings or progressions, prove more taxing than sounds in isolation or with easy transitions. Complexity of transition increases with the number of adjustments necessary to proceed from one setting to the next. Hence 'ski' should be more difficult than 'seek', and 'friendly' poses more problems than 'fondue'.

Errors tend to be in the direction of simplification (that is, unmarking) of segments or sequences (Deal and Darley, 1972; Trost and Canter, 1974; Keller, 1984). Thus 'chair' may become 'dair', 'friendly' becomes 'fendy'. Occurrences of seemingly more complex productions are found, for example, what is heard as 'chable' for 'table' or 'dlambp' for 'lamb'.

The nature of derailments does not permit a straightforward summary. This stems partly from the contrast between use of group data, which submerges individual pictures, versus single-case studies. It stems from sampling data elicited at different stages of recovery (compare Shankweiler and Harris (1966) and Sands, Freeman and Harris (1978) for a longitudinal study of a patient). Naturally it varies according to severity and with the prominence of associated dysphasia. Argument over where AS ends and dysphasia begins, or whether the two really are separable, has also led to different data interpretations. The arguments for and against AS as a language (phonological) disorder are presented in Martin (1974); Martin and Rigrodsky (1974); Halpern, Keith and Darley (1976); Klich, Ireland and Weidner (1979); Buckingham (1979); Rosenbek, Kent and La Pointe (1984a); Roy and Square (1985).

Earlier reports also classified errors according to the perceptual categories, said to characterise AS. They were substitutions (cable for table); omissions (sick or tick for stick); additions (sitamap for stamp); distortions (fwater for water); perseverations (popatoe for potato); anticipations (Kichael for Michael); and metathesis (nifished for finished, dicso for disco). As with articulatory phonetic errors, wide discrepancies exist in the reported relative distribution of these from study to study. It has also been questioned whether the pattern is unique to AS, or is also reflected in dysphasia (compare Blumstein, 1973; Martin and Rigrodsky, 1974; Trost and Canter, 1974; Halpern, Keith and Darley, 1976; Klich, Ireland and Weidner, 1979).

While these discrepancies reflect the same underlying variables (pages 90 and 95) as for articulatory disturbance, there are also added problems. Is the use of /k/ for /m/ in Michael an anticipatory or substitution error? Is 'puy' for 'buy' a substitution or a distortion (of voice onset time or aspiration)? Do 'sitamap' for 'stamp' or 'sfwim' for 'swim' represent addition errors, or do the sounds perceived as apparent additions arise as extraneous sounds in the person's efforts to transfer from one articulatory setting to the next? In other words, where does distortion end and substitution, omission and addition begin? What is the relationship between alleged motor derailment and the phonological (sound) system of the language in errors of anticipation, perseveration and claimed substitutions?

In this way, the use of these perceptual error categories has introduced more confusion than necessary into what is essentially an expressive disorder. The use of even fairly narrow phonemic transcriptions has also led to many features inaudible to the 'naked ear' being missed.

Relying on these superficial error patterns has proved to be inconclusive in dividing AS from any kind of dysphasic phonological impairment, has offered little or no help in the search for explanatory descriptions and has not led to any reliable remediation techniques. Analyses in terms of articulatory phonetics has advanced thinking on the topic, but still left interpretation dependent on observations of the 'naked ear', even when relatively narrow transcriptions were utilised. Over recent years, more objective methods of measuring dyspraxic speech have helped answer many of the questions raised by earlier research and have permitted new insights to be made.

Instrumental Analyses of Apraxia of Speech

Spectrographic studies have confirmed the acoustic correlates of the slow speech of dyspraxics, showing it as resulting from prolonged articulation and abnormal syllable segregation (Kent and Rosenbek, 1983). These features are lost in simple phonetic transcription. Further, they demonstrated reduced variation in relative peak intensity across syllables, correlating with the tendency to mono-loudness. Spectrographic recording also confirmed slow, inaccurate movements in vowel and consonant production. Vowel distortion, which to the naked ear is perceived to be relatively rare, was shown to be a common feature. Perceived voicing errors could be seen to arise from mistiming on voice onset and termination. The false starts, restarts and distortions are also shown up clearly in spectrographic analysis.

These are even clearer in electromyographic (EMG) investigation. Shankweiler, Harris and Taylor (1968) found abnormal EMG traces in their two dyspraxics, with marked variation in timing of sequential movements between articulators on repeated trials of the same task. Their recordings underlined the problems of independent movement of individual articulators.

Fromm, Abbs, McNeil *et al.* (1982) approached their EMG study of three relatively pure AS patients adopting a multi-level motor equivalence control model, as opposed to the previous level-by-level quasi-linear speech production model. They believed that utterances judged perceptually or spectrographically to be equivalent (that is, both normal or both distorted in the same manner) might be arrived at by motorically quite different paths. Their findings not only demonstrated this, offering EMG correlations to the disco-ordination and struggle perceived visually or acoustically, but they also highlighted features not accessible to acoustic analysis.

They were able to demonstrate considerable abnormal EMG activity preparatory to initiation of utterances and during apparent silences. What had been deemed distortion, addition or substitutions in traditional terminology were clearly related to neuro-muscular dysfunction. Their subjects evidenced antagonistic muscle contraction, continuous undifferentiated EMG activity, muscle activity shutdown, movement without voice, movement disco-ordination, addition and groping. Ninety-five per cent of all the substitution and addition errors in their study were produced with accompanying motor abnormalities. They were abnormalities distinct both from normal speakers' patterns and those of various dysarthric types previously studied.

Itoh and co-workers (Itoh, Sasanuma and Ushijima, 1979; Itoh, Sasanuma, Hirose *et al*., 1980; Itoh and Sasanuma, 1984) have used fiberscopic and X-ray microbeam observations to compare the movements of the velum and lower lip, the lower incisors and the tip and dorsum of the tongue in relation to each other and to the acoustic aspects of speech. They also compared these movements in AS patients with normal people and patients with other sound-patterning difficulties. Their findings demonstrated how acoustically similar, even apparently correct, sounds were produced with varying and abnormal movements. Itoh and Sasanuma concluded (1984, p. 158) that 'an articulatory disorder that is distinct from both asphasia and dysarthria can occur . . . and this disorder reflects malfunctions at the level of the motor programming of the articulators'. This is in opposition to those who would consider a predominantly, or exclusively, phonological disorder to be underlying dyspraxic speech.

Keatley and Pike (1976) underline that AS is not a disorder affecting solely the primary articulators. They assessed respiratory function and found it related to the severity of AS. In particular, four of their five patients had below normal peak expiratory flow.

Localisation

Statements on brain areas associated with AS have all been made with the caveats needed in assuming discrete anatomical sites correlate with behavioural manifestations. Traditionally, lesions to the third left frontal convolution, the area of secondary motor cortex linked with facial movement (also termed Broca's area) have been associated with AS (Mohr *et al*., 1978; Deutsch, 1984a; Marquardt and Sussman, 1984). However, Marquardt and Sussman's findings were equivocal in correlating clinical measures of AS and lesion site and size. It is well documented that lesions can occur to Broca's area without persisting speech and language sequelae (Mohr *et al*., 1978). Square and Mlcoch (1983), and Kertesz (1984) recorded cases of AS-like symptoms in left subcortical lesions. Typically, these involved either/or a combination of the putamen, globus pallidus, caudate nucleus, thalamus and the anterior and posterior limbs of the internal capsule. Lesions restricted to the striatal structures often showed less severe dysphasia, but AS was scarcely distinguishable from AS in cortical lesions.

So far the speech dyspraxic can be said to have difficulty in consistently realising speech sounds. Sometimes they say a sound or word correctly, and other times they do not. Speakers can often be seen to be struggling to get the right placements of lips, tongue and so on, which are eluding them even though primary muscle tone, power, co-ordination and sensation are adequate, and even though they can produce the same sound or word perfectly normally another time. To the listener it sounds as if the dyspraxic is omitting, distorting, substituting and mixing up the order of sounds. Instrumental analysis has demonstrated neuromuscular and acoustic correlates to these features.

The following sentence gives an overall impression of what AS might sound like. It is a rough transcription into normal English spelling of a person trying to say, 'In the summer they sell vegetables'. (The stress pattern is marked by ' and pauses by . . .). The reader is advised to say it aloud and listen to (1) how the flow is broken up by the pauses (during which the woman was struggling to find the correct placement of her articulators); (2) the abnormal stress patterning; (3) the distortion of sounds; and (4) the contrast between the slow, effortful, distorted main sentence and the perfectly normally spoken asides: 'Inn tsthe 'sumb . . . 'sub'ber . . . 'summ . . oh god . . . they 'zell . . . 'in the 'sumber 'dey 'se . . 'fedl . . . 'wara . . 'rowv . . , , 've . . 'xga . . 'ds'u . . 'g . . 'a. 'blsh . . I'm worse than I ever was.'

Having established a general picture of AS in speaking and on instrumental analysis, the performance of AS patients on assessment batteries and how it differs from other disorders will now be considered.

Assessment

While it seems clear from the studies reported so far that instrumental techniques are destined to play a leading role in the objective assessment of AS, currently these approaches are available only in experimental centres. Elsewhere, clinicians still have to rely on observational and analytical skills made with their own ear and eye, however misleading these have proved to be.

Clinical data comes from recordings of patients' spontaneous utterances and responses to stimuli designed to elicit the behaviours agreed to be indicative of AS. These are transcribed to the best of the clinician's ability in as narrow a transcription as possible, and errors are analysed from this.

There exist some semi-formal and formal procedures, for example,

Darley *et al.* (1975); Dabul (1979); and Wertz *et al.* (1984). These provide a framework and material for assessment, but interpretation of results is non-standardised and is made in relation to findings from the literature. As with other dyspraxia batteries reported here, the precise lexical and action content is not so vital. However, it is essential to include the main parameters of variation known to exist in dyspraxic speech, and between AS and other types of pronunciation deficit.

Single Consonant–Vowel Syllables

The syllables commonly chosen are /pa/, /ta/ and /ka/. The clinician listens for initiation ability, ability to maintain the integrity of the syllable over multiple, fast repetitions, and the nature of any derailments that do occur. Inconsistency of realisation (for example, drifting of /pa/ to /ta/ or what is heard as /ba/) or inability to sustain the sequence despite adequate breath and muscle power would be suggestive (though not pathognomic) of AS. Typically, the vowel is unstable as well as the consonant.

Multiple Syllable Repetition

The syllables used are usually /pa-ta-ka/, /ta-ka/ or /pa-ka/. One listens for disruptions to order, contamination between syllables, consistency of realisation, perseveration, anticipation, dysfluency of rhythm, ability to maintain the activity and skill at restarting after the sequence or sounds have been derailed. The 'apraxia of language' patients (p. 107) have little difficulty repeating single syllables, but on sequences may display ordering difficulties. They show no signs of struggle and flow is smooth and regular, only being disrupted by endeavours to regain the required sequence. The AS sufferer, if anything more than mild, will show errors of consistency, rhythm, silent and verbal struggle, and difficulty regaining patterns on single syllable repetition; severe cases may not get beyond one syllable. On sequential repetition, there are added problems of perseveration and inter-syllable contamination (compare Mateer and Kimura, 1977; Guyard, Sabouraud and Gagnepain, 1981). There may be considerable associated facial and body movement besides the verbal groping.

Articulatorily Simple and Complex Words

Complexity is a function of single segment composition (ch versus t), consecutive segment demands (sa versus sk), and overall length of word. Wertz *et al.* (1984) encourage their patients to say words such as 'gingerbread', 'artillery', 'snowman', 'responsibility', 'several', and 'statistical analysis'. It is also practice to compare multiple repetition of these words to monitor consistency of correctness and error, ease of flow from segment to segment, uniformity of stress and intonation features.

Because AS patients are said to experience growing difficulty with longer words, all assessment batteries have devised sets of words increasing in length, for example, 'thick-thicken-thickening'; 'flat-flatten-flattening' (Wertz *et al.*, 1984).

Sentence Reading and Repetition

These tasks are utilised to tax milder cases and observe loci of errors, for example, word initial, medial or final; content versus function words; common versus infrequent items; predictable versus less predictable sequences. AS people are more likely to show errors on word initial sounds in uncommon content words. Darley *et al.* (1975) use among their sentences: 'The shipwreck washed up on the shore'; 'Please put the groceries in the refrigerator.' The sentence repetition tasks in the Boston Diagnostic Aphasia Examination (Goodglass and Kaplan, 1983) are also ideal here.

Meaningful versus Meaningless Syllables

AS patients as a group are worse on meaningless strings. This is different from dysarthrics who tend to score equally on both types.

Spontaneous Speech Sample

This is gathered not only to observe segmental error types over larger stretches and to monitor prosody, speed and fluency, but also to listen for islands of clear speech, especially on asides, stereotyped phrases and over-learned material. It also offers the opportunity to observe associated body movements, respiration and awareness of errors.

Spontaneous, propositional production can also be compared to automatised expression, such as counting, days of the week, and completing proverbs or lines of well-known songs or prayers.

Reading and repeating sentences and extensive spontaneous speech may not be possible where a prominent dysphasia accompanies the AS. Procedures for distinguishing dyspraxic and dysphasic manifestations are mentioned below.

Oral Non-verbal Assessment

Although the causal relationship between oral dyspraxia and mispronunciations is unclear, an oral non-verbal examination is routinely carried out. Many workers include non-verbal oral work in the rehabilitation of verbal dyspraxia and so it is important to ascertain the level of any oral dyspraxia (Chapter 2). An oral physical assessment will also supply information on the extent of muscle tone, power and co-ordination deficit to the suspected AS. The degree of non-verbal oral function usually correlates directly with articulatory deficit in dysarthia, but not in AS.

Edwards (1984) has reviewed studies that do not support a direct correlation between speech and non-speech movements in dysarthrics. The studies covered, though, deal with the relationship of sucking, chewing, biting and swallowing to speech, rather than to muscle tone, power, co-ordination and diadochokinetic rates, which one would expect to have a more direct connection.

Oral Sterognosic Tests

These are also sometimes advocated. Some kind of tactile, kinaesthetic, proprioceptive feedback is essential for the efficient functioning of the speech system (see Borden, 1979). The exact nature and functioning of a feedback (and feed-forward) mechanism(s) is a matter of debate (Kelso and Tuller, 1981). Findings from studies covering this area in AS are mixed — some AS patients do have difficulty, others do not (Mateer and Kimura, 1977).

The significance of findings is difficult to evaluate because of the problems in measuring oral stereognosis. Two point discrimination on the lips or tongue and oral form identification and discrimination are far from the skills required in ongoing speech production. Furthermore, oral exploration demands, however minimal, a motor response as well as sensory exploration and integration. Deutsch (1981) found AS patients scored below normal people on oral stereognosis, but failed to distinguish them from dysphasics' scores in other studies, and did not establish a link between oral form identification and severity of speech production. Procedures and issues in oral stereognosis have been reviewed by Deutsch (1984b).

Auditory Discrimination

These tests have also been included in some studies of AS. It has not been shown to play a direct role in the misarticulations of AS (Square, Darley and Sommers, 1981). However, as sound monitoring and greater reliance on it are often emphasised in rehabilitation, it may be useful to exclude any marked auditory perceptual disorder.

Limb Dyspraxia Assessment

Thinking forward to possible rehabilitation strategies, the level, if any,

of limb dyspraxia (Chapter 2) can be gauged, especially if a manual sign-
ing system is going to be introduced to support or supplant spoken
language.

Language Evaluation

This is vital, as it aids in differential diagnosis. AS is most often associated
with Broca's (agrammatic), global and transcortical motor (Goodglass
and Kaplan, 1983) dysphasias. Apraxia of language (p. 107) is more
often linked with conduction and Wernicke's dysphasias. Dysarthria does
not generally co-occur with a significant degree of dysphasia.

The language assessment will also give indications of how far a person's lack of expressive speech might be due to AS and how much to
co-existing dysphasia. One could not expect fluent, grammatically well-
formed expression with severe receptive and expressive dysphasia, nor
with moderately good comprehension but moderate to severe Broca's
or transcortical motor dysphasia. Language assessment will also establish
how far word finding or retrieval difficulties might be contributing to
the poor expressive picture.

The level of language functioning will also be important in rehabilitation. It will perhaps need therapy before the AS. It will also set limits
on how much advance to expect in AS therapy and the efficacy of any
alternative means of communication. In general, the greater the language
involvement, the poorer the prognosis.

The language assessment should not neglect reading and graphic skills.
Some AS sufferers are assisted in their verbal expression by seeing the
written word, which may be helpful in later therapy, as well as for the
person's morale in communicating in general. Likewise, especially where
the dysphasia is minimal and AS not so severe, written expression is
often easier than spoken (see Figure 4.1). Unfortunately, the concomitant dysphasia usually precludes exploiting reading and writing as viable
alternatives.

Functional Communication

Alongside inspection of formal language skills, assessment of functional
communication provides information for intervention suitability. People
show a marked variation in what they are able to achieve with the skills
available to them. Two people with identical profiles on formal testing
may perform quite differently owing to their varying abilities to capitalise
on and mobilise what residual function they do have. Severe dysphasia
or AS rating does not necessarily equal severe communicative disorder.

Differential Diagnosis

The main areas of confusion in diagnosing AS arise in differentiating it from dysarthric speech, from non-motor dysphasic speech disorders and other language or intellectual dysfunction.

Apraxia of Speech and Dysarthria

These disorders represent breakdown at different levels of speech production: AS at a higher cortical level of organisation, dysarthria within the primary motor cortex, subcortical structures and pathways, and in the peripheral nervous system or in muscle function.

In general, the dysarthric person experiences problems in all oral activities (eating, swallowing, breathing), as well as speech, which is in keeping with the primary motor deficit. There may be exceptions, particularly in upper motor neurone type dysarthria. AS affects speech only. Apart from a right facial weakness, AS patients have normal facial gestures, while the Parkinsonian dysarthric, for instance, may display the typical poker face; and the motor neurone disease or myasthenia patient will have a facial expression associated with overall reduced muscle tone.

The possible associated motor deficits of AS are oral and limb dyspraxia and usually a (right) hemiplegia. Otherwise, range and speed of oral and limb movements are normal. According to dysarthric type, there may be generalised hyper- or hypotonus, ataxia, loss of full range of movement (for example, of the tongue or lip seal), decreasing excursion on alternating movements and festination.

AS is commonly found with agrammatic and global dysphasia, and less commonly with other dysphasic syndromes. Generally, dysarthrics have intact lexical and syntactic functioning. Where dysphasia and dysarthria do co-occur (Rosenbek, McNeil, Teetson *et al.*, 1981; Damasio, Damasio, Rizzo *et al.*, 1982; Naeser, Alexander, Helm-Estabrooks *et al.*, 1982), apart from in spastic (upper motor neurone) dysarthria, the dysphasic pictures are outside the traditionally identified syndromes. The exceptions to this are, naturally, in cases of multiple CVA or extensive head injury.

The speech characteristics most prominent in AS are: the inconsistency of realisation of segments and strings; islands of fluency, especially on asides, and automated sequences; frequent real and apparent substitutions, additions, perseveration and anticipation errors; and signs of articulatory struggle not related to muscle weakness. Increased effort in speech brings no significant or consistent improvement.

Conversely, dysarthrics present: a comparative homogeneity of errors, with predominantly distortions; no islands of clarity; struggle clearly derived from endeavours to counteract muscle weakness; and clear improvement gained from heightened attention and effort. There is little, if any, attempt to correct errors. To some degree or other, all aspects of speech will be disordered — respiration, voice, resonance, articulation — giving disorders of loudness, pitch, intonation and oral-nasal resonance balance. AS is essentially restricted to articulatory faults, and prosodic disturbance secondary to these and attempted corrections (Darley *et al.*, 1975; Kent and Rosenbek, 1982; Hartman, 1984). In dysarthria, word-class (content versus function) and frequency have little effect compared to AS.

When AS and dysarthria co-occur from a single lesion, it is usually a type of spastic dysarthria from involvement of the primary motor cortex and adjacent white matter. The dysarthric speech component is then analogous to the limb-kinetic disturbances (p. 40) that can accompany ideomotor dyspraxia.

Apraxia of Speech and Dysphasia

Wertz *et al.* (1984) report from previous data that dysphasia and/or dysarthria co-occur with AS in as many as 88 per cent of communication-disordered patients. Therefore, the clinical problem will more likely be the relative bearing of the two disorders on the person's communication difficulties, rather than a straightforward 'Is it A or B?' question. Dysphasics do exist without any articulation or phonological dysfunction, as do AS patients with negligible dysphasia.

Halpern, Darley and Brown (1973) administered various tasks to different groups of neurologically impaired people, among them speech dyspraxics and dysphasics. Several measures showed a tendency to differentiate these two groups.

Dysphasics scored significantly worse on auditory retention and naming. They were also poorer than the dyspraxics on writing to dictation, and syntax and fluency tasks. But with respect to these last-named tasks, while dysphasics scored worse than the dyspraxics, it should be noted that within the dyspraxic group itself these tasks received among the highest error scores. Thus, while dyspraxics are better at them than dysphasics, the prominence of errors in these areas is a pointer to dyspraxia.

On overall functioning capability, the dysphasic group rated more than twice as poorly as the AS group. This data is for relatively clearly divided AS and dysphasic groups.

The greater the discrepancy between comprehension level and expressive deficit, especially with evidence of articulatory errors, the more one should suspect AS. Good listening, reading and writing, but poor speaking suggests a profile of AS. The ability to indicate a desired word in writing or by pointing to alternatives, despite being unable to say it, supports a diagnosis of AS rather than dysphasia, where word finding may be a marked feature.

AS may be present, of course, in the context of moderate or severe comprehension loss; but then the distinction is more an academic exercise and not so relevant to the pressing clinical needs of coping with the comprehension loss and introducing any kind of communication, spoken or not.

Conduction Dysphasia

This is a disorder with which AS has traditionally been compared (Goodglass and Kaplan, 1983; Hécaen and Albert, 1978). It is characterised by fluent, effortless speech, with normal speed, stress and intonation. If speed is affected, it is in the direction of press of speech, rather than in slowness. Transition from one segment to another within and between words is normal. Breaks in flow come either from word-finding difficulties, or in attempts to correct pronunciation errors.

These latter errors show a characteristic pattern, which are similar to AS on the surface. They are: substitutions of one sound (phoneme) for another; omissions; additions; and disruption in sequencing (anticipation, perseveration, metathesis) across syllables and words.

The phonological make-up of the word(s) in error always follows the phonotactic rules of the language, that is, sequences of sounds within syllables do not occur that would not be permissible according to the rules of the language, such as 'gda', 'yeshch' and 'fpi' in English. Normally, the errors can be traced to factors within the *sound* environment (as opposed to movement or articulatory complexity). In mild cases, patients are generally aware of these derailments and attempt to correct them. In severer cases, especially in cases of Wernicke's dysphasia, no attempt might be made to rectify faults, thus resulting in words or stretches of neologistic jargon.

The efforts to self-correct in the milder cases bring about *conduites d'approche*, whereby the person makes repeated attempts at saying a word in order to gain the right pronunciation. The succession of tries does not proceed step by step nearer the target and the person, having chanced upon the desired production, might as easily again lose it. This example from personal data is of a man trying to say 'carpet': 'Ter . . .

ter . . . terbak . . . der . . . derpak . . . terpak . . . ter . . . ter . . .
tar . . . terpet . . . terpot . . . ter . . . terpet . . . terpet . . . ter . . .
ter . . . terpit . . . terpit . . . cherpik . . . terpet . . . tarpet . . . carpot
. . . sharket . . . sharket . . . sharkitit . . . shar . . . no, sher . . . a
ter . . . kerpet . . . car . . . carpet.'

Several features have led to conduction dysphasia being considered
a disorder of sound system programming, and not one of motor execution. These include: the effortless performance; the integrity of the
phonotactic (sound combination) rules; the relative accuracy in single
sound production compared to disordered sequential performance; and
the phonemic (errors across class) as opposed to phonetic (distortions
within class) nature of sound errors.

Thus, it contrasts with AS where speech is effortful and slowed; where
sounds or combinations of sounds are heard that are atypical of the
language; where single sound production is disordered and sequential
production is frequently marked by strong tonic perseveration; and where
sound errors are predominantly of phonetic distortion.

This dichotomy, here drawn between conduction dysphasia and AS,
has been confirmed under numerous other headings as distinguishing
between an anterior, executive type disorder and a posterior breakdown
in planning.

Luria (1973) spoke of afferent motor dysphasia for the higher order
type, and efferent motor dysphasia for the lower order, production type
disorder. Derouesne, Beauvois and Ranty (1977), supporting Luria,
expressed the same division in terms of paradigmatic, selectional and
syntagmatic, combinational, error types. Guyard, Sabouraud and Gagnepain (1981) found similar criteria distinguished between the speech of
Wernicke's and Broca's dysphasics. Mackenzie (1982) provided data
reflecting the same contrast under the labels 'aphasic phonological' and
'aphasic articulatory' defect. Nespoulous, Lecours and Joanette (1983)
examined the validity of the distinction in terms of phonemic (literal
paraphasic, higher order) versus phonetic errors. Buckingham (1983)
speaks of apraxia of language versus apraxia of speech.

Square *et al.* (1982) reported that differing lesion sites may give differing speech characteristics in pure(r) speech dyspraxic patients. Deutsch
(1984a) confirmed predictions by Luria (1973) and others, that fluent
'apraxia of language' errors are associated with left posterior lesions,
while dysfluent, effortful speech production was more often linked with
anterior lesions.

Damasio and Damasio (1980) studied the anatomical basis of conduction dysphasia. In their series of six patients, five showed compromise

or left insula and variable degree of involvement of the superior temporal gyrus and an extension into inferior parietal area. The lesions were deep in all cases, involving the white matter subjacent to the above regions. No cases involved angular gyrus nor Broca's area.

This distinction finds parallels in other dyspraxias. Mateer and Kimura (1977), Ohigashi *et al.* (1980) and Watamori *et al.* (1981) found it in oral dyspraxia. Kimura (1977, 1982) and Roy (1981, 1983) describe it in limb dyspraxias. The constant, which binds these studies, appears to indicate a posterior (temporal–parietal) role in higher level assembling of programmes, and an anterior (frontal, opercular) role in execution. Buckingham's (1983) term 'apraxia of language' would seem well chosen as a parallel to the posterior limb dyspraxias that produce the parapraxic substitutions and part-substitutions, as opposed to the anterior distortions and inertia of response.

Results from these studies also indicate that the division is not a strict either–or, but, according to lesion site and extent, a tendency towards one or the other extreme. Keller (1984) further corroborates this. His conduction dysphasics showed some definite AS errors; his Broca's dysphasics showed evidence of dysarthric errors, presumably akin to the limb-kinetic errors (p. 40) of limb dyspraxics.

Conduction dysphasia, of course, is not diagnosed just on the basis of literal paraphasic errors. They are part of a broader picture including anomia, dysgrammatism, comprehension loss, auditory perceptual deficits and reading and writing problems.

Therapy for Apraxia of Speech

This section deals with aspects of dyspraxia therapy more specific to AS. A general discussion of dyspraxia therapy is covered in Chapter 8. Clearly, these brief paragraphs could not do justice to the scope and detail of intervention in AS, which would require an extensive, independent work. Such a thorough work has been published, in fact, by Wertz *et al.* (1984). Broadly, approaches can be categorised into those that are direct and indirect. The former tackle the motor speech disorder head on, the latter facilitate communication either through techniques that enable the sufferers themselves to bypass the central problem, or by creating a communicative environment that minimises the handicap created by AS and maximises compensation through the person's strengths.

Counselling

Counselling is an essential feature of all therapy. It is as important for the family and friends to know about the disorder and prospects as much as it is for the patient. While speech is still inadequate, everyone needs to know how best to understand the dyspraxic's feelings and ideas, especially if written expression is not possible and the person is unable to manage a communication chart or mechanical substitute. Such patients may need to be made aware of the concept of total communication, something of which they were not aware before; this includes non-verbal clues such as facial expression, posture gesture, routine and context.

The nature of AS should be described to everyone who is involved. They should be told the significance of islands of fluency and of words being pronounced well 'out of the blue', but which are not possible later on; and the reason for well-articulated swear words but poorly articulated family names; and the fact that such variation is not a sign of obstinacy, laziness, negativism or dementia on the part of the dyspraxic. It is the therapist's duty to instruct people about how best they can facilitate responses from the dyspraxic — through careful phrasing of the question to demand answers within the person's capability; through structuring of the environment to allow alternative means of comprehension and expression and to minimise competing, distracting, overloading or hindering practices and stimulation.

The question of day-to-day variation needs elaborating: dyspraxics like everyone else experience on and off days but, for them, added fatigue, tension or depression can make the difference between efficient and failed verbal performance. Families must be helped to cope with failure from this and other sources.

In rehabilitation, the role of the therapist, dyspraxic, the family and others requires clear delineation. The family must have realistic goals and expectations as much as anyone else. They must understand the constant commitment demanded for therapy and the gradual nature of improvement. As yet, there are no magic pills or operations to restore immediately bilabial plosives or high-back vowels. It is vital that everyone concerned must appreciate that at some stage formal therapy will cease, and that the dyspraxic patient will, most likely, still be far from the verbal wizard they once were.

Alas, limited space precludes a proper discussion of counselling in AS here. A sympathetic and detailed exposition of the area appears in Wertz *et al.* (1984). Florance, Rabidoux and McCauslin (1980), Newhoff, Florance, Malone *et al.* (1980) and Lubinski (1981) provide practical discussion.

Direct Therapy

For severe AS, direct therapy has proceeded traditionally on a sound-by-sound basis (Rosenbek, Lemme, Ahern *et al.*, 1973; Dabul and Bollier, 1976; Deal and Florance, 1978), starting with the easiest. This is decided for the individual either from results of ease of imitation, or if no clear-cut order exists, then on the basis of articulatory simplicity. These are combined with factors of visibility and commonness in the language. The look-and-listen pattern of progression, often coupled with tactile and manipulative stimulation of the articulators, is a habit established from the start.

In very difficult circumstances, articulatory gestures have been preceded by nonverbal oral exercises and production has been broken down into its component parts — for example, biting bottom lip, expiring air through the constriction, and then adding voice to produce /v/. Since co-ordination of the various components for sounds and incorporation of them into syllables and words is precisely the problem encountered in AS, it seems intuitively disadvantageous to dwell long at this stage. Unfortunately, it is often necessary in severe cases.

An approach that introduces sounds in context and sounds with meaning as soon as possible is more favourable both for communicative ability and for the patient's morale — not to mention the therapist's. In this respect, contrasting sounds are introduced as soon as feasible (vowels as well as consonants). Where possible, syllables are used that form real words — either on their own (my, buy, pea, tea), or later, when combined build multisyllable words (to-day, tea-V).

The words chosen are preferably common words with a strong emotive or associative tie, that are going to be of immediate use to the person. Maximum use is made of residual skills on, for example, automatic sequences. Numbers and letters give 'B-4' for 'before'; 'want' can be derived from 'one' t(wo)'; 'fried egg' from 'Friday', and so on. The length of phrase can be extended by tapping stereotyped phrases, or lines of songs that may be more accessible than isolated words. These act as carrier phrases or lead-ins for other words. Hill (1978) provides extensive detail of the kinds of words and phrases clinicians use to elicit isolated sounds or syllables, and to build up multisyllable words and phrases.

Early on, it is good for morale to encourage use of residual words, or fragments of words, and to create quasi-conversation. In this, the able speaker structures the conversation with the AS person to elicit intact phrases ('good morning', 'fine day', 'no thanks') or lead into retrained words with associated entrances. 'Have you had your breakfast?'; 'Did you get a cup of ——?'; 'Can I help you put on your shoes and ——?'

Stress and intonation become topics of rehabilitation with milder dyspraxics, who can utter short phrases. Control of proper stress and intonation can have a beneficial effect on intelligibility, even without a parallel improvement in articulatory precision. Contrasting stress patterns can be used to signal changes of meaning in phrases such as '*That*'s my coat' versus 'That's *my* coat' versus 'That's my *coat*'. Intonation can be exploited also to assist the person in making his limited expressive efforts go further — 'That's right' or 'Yours' said with a statement versus an interrogative intonation.

Melodic intonation therapy successfully employed with dysphasics has also been advocated in AS (Tonkovich and Marquardt, 1977). It is said to facilitate initiation and fluency, but it also aids prosodic features.

Spoken language will not be a realistic goal for some people. Alternative or augmentative means of communication must be considered then. Dowden, Marshall and Tompkins (1981) utilised Amer-Ind sign language as a facilitator of verbalisation. From personal experience, Blissymbolics (Archer, 1977) have also proved effective. Rabidoux, Florance and McCauslin (1980) successfully introduced the 'Handivoice' machine to three severe dyspraxics.

Suitability for non-speech methods must be evaluated in the context of the environmental demands made on the person's communication (how many more people will have to be taught the system?; how portable is it?); the person's non-dyspraxic deficits, such as hemiplegia or ideomotor dyspraxia (see page 35–6 on novel learning); and, most importantly, dysphasia severity. The scope for other means of communication is seriously restricted if there is significant language deficit. Motivation and adaptability of the patient and his family, likewise, are decisive.

Prognosis

Statements here relate chiefly to improvement in spoken communication and not in overall functional communication. Commonly, the two are quite separate. An understanding of extra-linguistic variables that may have a bearing (age, intellect, motivation, onset of rehabilitation, environmental support) is taken as read. Wertz's (1984) finding of higher non-verbal intelligence (Raven's progressive matrices) scores linked with those patients who improved significantly deserves special mention among these factors.

It is difficult to extricate dyspraxic from dysphasic prognostic indicators in considering speech and language variables. Wertz (1984) showed that the two can recover at varying rates, and that change in one was not linked significantly to change in the other. Initial severity of AS, among his subjects, did not relate significantly to initial severity of dysphasia. AS patients who improved did so by one or two points on his seven-point severity scale, irrespective of whereabouts on the scale they started.

However, clinicians will recognise instances where accompanying marked dysphasia has been associated with poor prognosis in AS. This is the case where comprehension loss is considerable. Valuable time and effort needs to be expended on rehabilitation in that area, and AS therapeutic techniques are restricted by the concomitant underlying language problem. It is also true in the case where poor comprehension precludes effective monitoring of errors. Non-awareness of errors is a poor omen for improvement. Likewise, marked transcortical motor (adynamic) dysphasia sets limits on expressive improvement, where, despite good performance to external cues, the person remains unable to initiate utterances themselves. The reports of Hill (1978) are typical in this respect.

Mohr *et al.* (1978) indicated that a lesion restricted to Broca's area (third left frontal convolution) — their so-called 'little or minor Broca's syndrome' — was associated with favourable prognosis, while more extensive lesions ('big Brocas'), which had accompanying language difficulties, had a poorer outlook.

The influence of oral dyspraxia on AS therapy outcome is not that it directly impedes progress, but that the range of effective therapy options is curtailed by its presence. The existence of a significant dysarthric component in the pronunciation disability does not directly inhibit improvement in the AS. However, it does constitute an area that may require additional therapy and may mask underlying AS improvement.

Patients who are going to get better without therapy do so within days, or weeks at the most. All others must rely on their own and the therapist's dedicated application to gain advance. The longer the period of initial mutism, the bleaker the prospects.

If there are arguments concerning many aspects of AS theory and therapy, one feature that finds consensus is the intensity and length of commitment required in AS therapy. The minimum is daily application, with less than that being tantamount to providing no therapy at all. Even with this, one envisages therapy in terms of months for mild debilitation, years for moderate debilitation, and indefinitely in cases of severe AS and marked dysphasia. This underlines the importance of total commitment on the part of the dyspraxic and his family, and of their ability to take over responsibility for carrying out exercises and techniques. It also emphasises the centrality of correct counselling from the rehabilitation team in helping the individual, family and friends to make this adjustment. Prognosis is poor where sufficient motivation for such involvement cannot be achieved or sustained.

Wertz (1984) concludes that individual direct therapy begun as soon as possible produces better results than group therapies. Other positive indicators in treatment are the attainment and maintenance of therapeutic goals, and the generalisation of skills relearned. The saw-tooth profile of progress, where advance is made in one session, only to have to be started from scratch again in the next, is a poor sign. Inability to generalise learning also bodes ill; for example, if the person has learned lip closure for /p/ and then has to learn it anew for /b/.

Despite an overall optimistic impression from the literature and clinical experience, all clinicians will know of patients who have failed to respond to even the best planned and executed therapy. These patients tend to be those with marked associated comprehension loss; associated written expressive deficit; poor awareness of errors; reluctance to, or inability to, apply themselves independently to therapy; and those who show no generalisation or retention in therapy. The role of the therapist as counsellor assumes added importance in such cases, the person must not simply be rejected on to a scrap-heap of the neurologically impaired. The ability of the rehabilitation team and family to create an optimally suitable environment is also called upon even more urgently in these instances. Wertz *et al.* (1984) and the other sources provided for counselling cover this area most ably.

Conclusion

A disorder has been described that is a dyspraxia in as far as: (1) it affects volitional as opposed to automatic movements; (2) it is a disorder of movement not explainable on the basis of defects in primary motor-sensory functioning; (3) there are characteristic error types related to disruption of volitional motor programming; and (4) instrumental measures have corroborated these underlying problems. In the patterns of errors and qualitatively different types according to site of lesion, it can be compared to parallel breakdowns in other dyspraxic pictures.

However, in its closeness to language production — in a broader sense rather than simply movements for the speech sounds of language — a full appreciation of the manifestations of AS involves consideration of other linguistic parameters. In this respect, a comparison was drawn with constructional dyspraxia, the full appreciation of which demands reference to the visual–perceptual processes that underlie motor execution.

5 OCULAR-MOTOR APRAXIA

Ocular-motor apraxia (OMA) is a disorder of horizontal voluntary movements of the eyes, in which patients are unable to direct their gaze as desired, although a full, random and involuntary range of movement exists. *A*praxia, as opposed to *dys*praxia, is used in this context merely because it is the term that has become established in the literature; it does not necessarily imply a complete absence of willed movement. An acquired and a congenital form have been described.

Congenital Ocular-motor Apraxia

The congenital or developmental form was first described as a separate clinical entity by Cogan (1952), and thus is sometimes called Cogan's syndrome. Another synonym is 'oculomotor apraxia', although this label can be objected to on the grounds that, strictly speaking, oculomotor disorder refers to a defect of the third cranial nerve only, rather than to eye movements in general. 'Dyspraxia of gaze' is a further synonym that has occurred in the literature.

The main presenting symptoms are:

1. Inability to voluntarily shift gaze horizontally;
2. Voluntary refixation accompanied by characteristic jerking of the head;
3. Normal vertical saccadic and pursuit movements;
4. Normal reflex movements of the eyes, except that;
5. Optokinetic nystagmus on horizontal strip or drum stimulation is absent or reduced.

Inability to Shift Gaze

While the child is randomly scanning its environment, eye movements in all directions are of normal range and speed. However, if the child already has his gaze fixed on something and is then required to switch fixation to a stimulus (visual or auditory) in the peripheral visual field or beyond, he is unable to do so; that is, there is an absence of voluntary horizontal saccades. In less marked cases, the child may be able to reach a target by means of a series of short saccades.

The defect is not restricted to saccadic movements. If an object passes

115

by in the child's horizontal plane, or an object on which the child has fixated begins to move sideways, the child is unable to follow it with his eyes, that is, there is absence of horizontal smooth pursuit. In less severe cases, tracking of slowly moving objects may be possible, and pursuit only fails at faster speeds. Some less severely affected children may be able to pursue objects by producing a string of short saccades.

For some children, there is an asymmetry of movement, with voluntary gaze being more difficult to one side than to the other (Cogan, 1966; Zee, Yee and Singer, 1977; Samson, Mihout, Proust and Parain, 1983). According to Zee *et al.*, the more volitional the task, the more severe the abnormality.

Head Jerks

A normal person wishing to switch the focus of attention usually starts by diverting the eyes and only afterwards turns the head. Head movement always lags behind eye movement. The latter is always adversive, that is, movement in the orbits is always in the same direction as the head turn. Movement of the eyes is commonly associated with a blink of the lids, a feature usually absent in the child with OMA. The turn of the head normally never overshoots the target. In brief fixation of an eccentric object in normal people, the head may not even be moved, or if it does move it is not turned fully towards the stimulus.

In contrast, a completely different strategy appears in OMA. In gaining voluntary (re)fixation, the child turns his head rapidly in the direction of the stimulus. However, because the child is unable to voluntarily move his eyes, this rotation of the head about its vertical axis results in a maintained contraversive deviation of the eyes, that is, eye movement lags behind head movement, and the eyes end up directed in the opposite sides of the orbits from which they should be. Therefore, to bring the new object into central vision the child must considerably overshoot the target with the head rotation until the eyes, in extreme contraversion, are dragged on to the target. Once the eyes have fixated the object, the head is then turned back towards it, with the eyes, remaining steadily centred on the target, being returned to their primary position in the orbits through the action of the vestibulo-ocular reflex. The whole cycle of head thrusting and refixation happens in less than a second.

Zee *et al.* (1977) presented some less severely affected patients who, when free to move their heads, did not show complete inability to refixate, but the children displayed defects of initiation closer to those described in more severe cases with the head immobilised.

Not all reports state when the head thrusts first arose in particular patients. Onset ranges from a few weeks after birth (Orrison and Robertson, 1979, case six) to the second year (Kaufmann, 1979) or even later (Rendle-Short, Appleton and Pearn, 1973). Mostly, it appears around six to nine months.

There has been some discussion as to whether the head-jerking represents an independent associated feature of OMA, or whether it is a compensatory strategy secondary to the difficulty with voluntary horizontal saccadic or pursuit movements. Zee *et al.* (1977) have reviewed the arguments and present experimental data from their own subjects, and compared it to the normal pattern of eye–head co-ordination. They concluded that the forceful thrusting and overshooting head movements were indeed part of an adaptive strategy to effect rapid changes in gaze. Interested readers are referred to this work for discussion of presumed underlying mechanisms and variations in strategy.

If head thrusting represents a compensatory strategy, and it varies in precise nature according to the level of intactness of the different ocular-motor mechanisms, then this might be one source of variation in age of onset of head jerking. The age at which infants start to use head jerks would depend on their ability to 'learn' the strategy and on the urgency to develop some method of voluntarily diverting their gaze (see also p. 124).

Vertical and Reflex Eye Movements

There is only one reported case of congenital OMA where vertical movements were said to be affected (Araie, Ozawa and Awaya, 1977). However, the patient presented with cerebellospinal degeneration, and hence the absence of vertical excursions cannot be taken unequivocally to be directly linked with the OMA.

There are no reports of cases with defects in pupillary reaction to light, convergence or vestibulo-ocular reflex. Indeed, some have pointed to the inability to suppress the vestibulo-ocular reflex as a causative factor in OMA. A frequent finding, though, is the absence of optokinetic nystagmus on horizontal strip or drum stimulation. Movement is completely abolished in many cases, while there may be some deviation in less severe instances, particularly at slow velocities. Typically though, the fast phase remains lacking.

Secondary Manifestations

Aside from the head jerking, if present, the most frequently observed behaviour directly associated with OMA concerns poor, or absent, performance on tasks that require intact voluntary saccadic and pursuit movement. Parents often feel that their child is blind in the first month of life. To them, he appears to stare blankly into space, to move his eyes around without purpose, and fails to pursue objects held up in front of him or to follow people across the room with his eyes. While he may be reacting to sudden noises, people entering the room or traffic passing by outside, he does not seem to be able to locate the source visually. Concern regarding visual acuity is a common reason for the child being brought to the health visitor or family doctor. Worries may be reinforced when behavioural visual acuity testing, for instance, employing a preferential-looking technique, fails to produce consistent results. The very difficulties faced by the OMA child preclude success on such tests. Gittinger and Sokol (1982) have circumvented this problem by testing for age-related normal acuity using pattern-reversal visual evoked responses.

Difficulties in locomotion are reported in changing direction, especially suddenly. The child, presumably being unable to scan the ground ahead, tends to misjudge openings and bumps into objects. Climbing and balancing on walls, horseback and tricycle riding, and following a thrown or bouncing ball are all reported problems. Nevertheless, many children appear to become adept at athletic activities in school and in later life. How far the reported hindrances are attributable to the ocular-motor deficits and how far they are associated with the commonly recorded motor difficulties is not entirely clear, and is a point considered later.

Another problem can arise on school entry. Reading acquisition is retarded owing to scanning difficulties. Children may be able to read single words but break down when obliged to read horizontal sequences and sentences. It is hard to establish whether reading difficulty is a constant finding in OMA. Many of the reported cases were too young to have started reading. Other children (for example, Orrison and Robertson, 1979, case one) were noted to have experienced retardation early on, but later were assessed as having normal reading skills. In others, the deficit would appear to persist into adulthood (Keiner and Keiner, 1958; Vassella, Lütschg and Mumenthaler, 1972).

Samson *et al.* (1983) speculate that many dyslexics may prove, on careful examination, to have subclinical forms of OMA. A further complicating factor in establishing a causative relationship between OMA and dyslexia is the frequent co-occurrence of the disorder with a language deficiency. The exact nature of the relationship is explored in more detail below.

Reading problems are not the sole area of difficulty on school entry even though they may be the most obvious. Much learning takes place through scanning pictures, blackboards, toys and the environment in general. The concepts of spatial relationships overall and their acquisition in the child depend on unimpaired visual input, not restricted solely to normal acuity.

Yarbus (1967) has detailed the nature of eye movements under various conditions, including in the perception of complex objects and pictures; during reading; for assessing spatial relationships; and in the appreciation of proportion, length, angles and area. Essential to an optimal performance in these tasks is an intactness of ocular control. Successful learning in these instances rests not only with the proper functioning of the muscular apparatus of the eye (thus those with a paralysis, as opposed to apraxia of gaze, also experience problems in this respect), but with the proper integration of the higher mental activity and voluntary eye movements.

Kephart (1971) and Ayres (1973) also emphasise the importance of intact ocular motor function in child development. The OMA child is handicapped in the exploration of and familiarisation with the visual-spatial world in the same way as the limb dyspraxic child is in its coming to terms with the tactile-perceptual-motor environment. Impaired ocular control affects the execution of certain actions and intentions formulated at higher cortical levels. But, in turn, it affects correspondingly the acquisition of the thought processes prerequisite to formulating the 'ideas'. Tyler (1969) has demonstrated defective eye movements in adult dysphasic patients and the consequences for comprehension of visual stimuli and expressive output regarding these.

Associated Disorders

Mental retardation (IQ < 75) is reported in approximately 14 of the 90 or so cases in the literature so far. The number is uncertain because not all histories detail mental development, and many patients are not of an age where reliable statements on mental development could be made.

Much more widespread are reports of OMA with motor and language delay. Only about 14 per cent of those who mention motor development say that it is normal. There is some kind of motor abnormality in the rest, ranging from mildly delayed motor milestones, a mild awkwardness and clumsiness in fine and/or gross movements, to more definite ataxia (the most commonly noted problem), general hypotonia (for example, Carecchi and Gainotti, 1977; Zee *et al.*, 1977, case three; Samson *et al.*, 1983, case one), and severe motor milestone delay.

Case three of Ferrer-Abizanda, Alvarez *et al.* (1977) achieved unsupported sitting only at two years of age, and unaided walking with broad-based gait at three and a half years, while his brother did not walk unsupported until he was four. Case seven of Orrison and Robertson (1979) sat unaided only at two years and was still unable to walk at three and a half years. Other writers have found spasticity and mild right hemiplegia (Cogan, 1952, case four), but such reports appear to be isolated, with the typical picture being delayed milestones and ataxia.

Like motor development, the degree of language handicap, when reported, ranges from none apparent, through mild delay, to marked deficiency (Ferrer-Abizanda *et al.*, 1977; Orrison and Robertson, 1979; Samson *et al.*, 1983). These patients are in addition to those who showed language delay as part of a general mental retardation, and to those who are reported to have had temporary or persisting difficulties with reading.

It is unclear to what extent the clumsiness, poor balance, awkward gait, delayed motor and language milestones share a common underlying cause(s) with OMA, and how far they are actually a result of the primary OMA difficulty. Dysfunction of the cerebellar pathways and the cerebellum itself have been implicated in OMA (see below). Such dysfunction could also be expected to compromise development of motor co-ordination and cause hypotonia, as well as to produce dysarthric speech. Other putative aetiologies of OMA, for example, some metabolic disorders, are also widely reported in the literature on motor and language delay as being possible causes of those problems.

On the other hand, intactness of visual input is a vital prerequisite in normal child development. Although the OMA child is not blind, one could justifiably describe him as partially sighted due to the restrictions on visual search and attention imposed by the dyspraxic condition. For this reason, many of the techniques and contents of intervention that have proved successful in maximising developmental progress in visually handicapped children, may be useful in minimising the negative effects of OMA on motor and linguistic advancement.

Like the OMA child, the partially sighted youngster does not have perfect balance, has poor motility, and impairment of visual guidance and judgement for fine and gross motor exploration, for monitoring success and failure visually, and hence for learning. These children, like OMA children, are reported to have poor estimation of tilt and poor righting reflexes under visual guidance. They experience a reduced, or lack of, awareness of motor potential for reaching in and exploring their environment visually from a static position, or actively under visual guidance. They are also handicapped in the acquisition of visual–auditory associations through their difficulty in turning to, and locating, sound sources.

Therapy

Therapeutic intervention, if deemed necessary, should be directed towards creating a learning environment where the disadvantages imposed by the OMA are anticipated, minimised or prevented. The returns from direct therapy on eye movements would not appear to warrant the amount of time that would need to be spent on them. The only mention in the literature of direct intervention (Cogan, 1952, 1966, case one) found that it is was unsuccessful.

As in most cases the condition remits spontaneously, it would seem more prudent to aim to give the child the same developmental input as his peers. In this way, when OMA is no longer a prime source of disability, one would hope that the child would be, as far as possible, on a par with his contemporaries in areas of visual perception, spatial exploration, auditory-visual awareness and the like, and not be left with a secondary set of handicaps to be tackled. Thus parents can be advised how to encourage correct posture and facilitate sitting, righting and motility. They can be shown how to help eye-hand, eye-foot and eye-body co-ordination. The shortfall in perceptual development through reduced visual input can be assisted by emphasising learning through the intact auditory and haptic channels. For those facing reading problems from OMA, Kaufmann (1979) recommends placing the book at right-angles to the person to capitalise on the intact vertical eye movements. As voluntary eye control is established, so books can be placed normally.

Space does not permit full details of all areas of therapy, nor of the techniques involved. Such information can be found in works dealing specifically with these areas, for example, Kephart (1971) and Ayres (1973).

Prognosis

No large-scale surveys of the long-term course of OMA exist. In fact, there is only one patient who has been followed into adulthood (Cogan, Chu, Reingold *et al.*, 1980). In 1966 Cogan reviewed his original (1952) patients, the two eldest being 19 years old by then. All other indications of prognosis to date are contained either in short-term reassessments (Orrison and Robertson, 1979), or are inferred from retrospective reports of patients first seen only at a late age (Keiner and Keiner, 1958; Cogan, 1966; Robles, 1966; Vassella *et al.*, 1972; Godel, Nemet and Lazar, 1979).

Cogan remarked in his 1952 description of the syndrome that it was of interest that the congenital form of the disorder was not observed in adults. The majority of reports that have pursued the fate of the abnormal eye and head movements into later childhood have reported a spontaneous gradual remission, with the ocular and associated (head thrusting, language and motor) symptoms no longer apparent by the first years at school. Those children who experience reading and writing difficulties and 'clumsiness' on school-entry integrate well into normal classes, have normal intelligence and attain age-appropriate performance in their subjects. Enduring handicaps appear to be linked with other incapacities — either frank motor disorders, as opposed to the minimal signs reported with OMA, or a generalised mental retardation (for example, Cogan, 1952, 1966, case four; Orrison and Robertson, 1979, case eight). Those cases that have shown deterioration all proved to have additional CNS complications (Lyle, 1961; Zaret, Behrens and Eggers, 1980).

However, difficulties in certain areas may last on into adulthood (Keiner and Keiner, 1958; Vassella *et al.*, 1972), despite the fact that the head jerks cease, voluntary horizontal eye movements are established and sufferers come to function normally to all intents and purposes, without need of any specific intervention. Persisting difficulties may resurface when the patient is under stress, fatigued (Cogan, 1966; Godel *et al.*, 1979) or in response to specific clinical tests.

The 34-year-old biologist reviewed by Cogan *et al.*, 1980 (case two of his 1952 group) was essentially asymptomatic, but admitted to some problems in tracking moving red blood cells under his microscope. He also reported that his eyes locked in place occasionally and at times he experienced head thrusts. This contrasted with completely inhibited eye movements and present but inconspicuous head thrusts at the age of 12 when he was engrossed in an object. He was proficient at the sports he chose (American football), but had had problems following the flight of the shuttlecock in badminton. Dancing posed some difficulties, and he experienced head thrusts particularly after some fast rotations. At the age of 19 he said he lost his balance easily, but this was not a significant drawback in his lifestyle at 34. He had always been an abnormally slow reader, despite taking 'speed-reading' courses, a point that would seem to lend support to the contention of Samson *et al.* (1983) that subclinical forms of OMA may contribute to reading problems in some people. Though other persisting abnormalities could be confirmed under laboratory conditions, the reports of his functional difficulties suggest that the abnormalities were not incapacitating.

OMA is not the only disorder in childhood presenting with abnormal saccades or atypical head movements. Taylor (1980) and Gresty, Halmagyi and Taylor (1983) have reviewed the various causes. Abnormal compensatory head movements, according to Taylor (1980), are only likely to occur with disorders of saccadic movement, since the loss of tracking ability in pursuit movement defects can be compensated for by using multiple saccades.

Cogan, Chu, Reingold and Barranger (1981) have discussed ocular motor signs in some metabolic disorders. Grover, Tucker and Wenger (1978) went as far as to term the ocular-motor abnormality they described in Gaucher's disease (glucocerebrosidase deficiency) 'dyspraxia of gaze'.

Ocular disturbances are also typical of over 80 per cent of ataxia telangiectasia sufferers, and the picture is close to that of OMA. Some writers have questioned whether or not some cases of OMA are early or incomplete cases of ataxia telangiectasia (Narbona, Crisci and Villa, 1980). Arthuis (1968) and Samson *et al.* (1983) argue against such a view, as do Baloh, Yee and Boder (1977). Most significant are that vertical movements are also involved, and that a target is always reached if a child is given sufficient time.

As regards the aetiology of OMA, many proposals have been made, but none has been conclusive. A genetic predisposing factor has been suggested by Rendle-Short *et al.* (1973) and Neetens and Rubbens (1982). The many cases of twins, siblings or succeeding generations being affected lends support to this view (Robles, 1966; Vassella *et al.*, 1972; Ferrer-Abizanda *et al.*, 1977; Godel *et al.*, 1979).

Orrison and Robertson (1979) speculated on a- or dysgenesis of the corpus callosum being responsible, and Narbona *et al.* (1980) favoured an immune deficiency explanation. Lyle (1961) and Zaret *et al.* (1980) are the only workers to report OMA in cases of neoplasm.

Another possibility is that congenital OMA is a matter not of any identifiable underlying disorder, but of straightforward maturational delay. The gradual, spontaneous remission of symptoms would be accounted for aptly by such a theory, as would the reappearance of symptoms when faced with more complex tasks (for example, reading or playing tennis), or under conditions of suboptimal performance (for example, fatigue or tension). Such patterns of remission and reappearance under certain circumstances are well documented in other areas of developmental delay. Children with developmental speech or language disorders that apparently disappear in childhood, might nevertheless be more susceptible to become dysfluent when fatigued or under stress, or experience persisting difficulties on highly verbal tasks, despite otherwise seeming to cope adequately.

'Dyspraxia' of eye movements is a normal state in the neonate, as is the dominance of particular primitive reflexes — for example, 'doll's-eyes' reflex and the 'cornering' reflex movement of the eyes to sudden auditory stimulus. Focal length in the newborn is about 25 to 30 centimeters, and adult ranges of acuity are normally present only by the second year. In the first two months of life, the infant will only fleetingly follow a ball dangled before the eyes at the correct focal distance. Gradually, this behaviour extends with the development of focal length and with the velocity at which the eyes are able to track. Efficient pursuit of objects and people is established at around six or seven months. It is also around this age that reaching and hand–eye co-ordination commence, as well as intent visual inspection of objects. The development of voluntary head and neck control, as well as increased perceptual awareness of the environment, must also play a role in the age of onset of overt symptoms.

It is probably not coincidental that in most patients who transpire to have OMA, it is at this stage that parents begin seriously to suspect that the child has (visual) problems and that the abnormal head jerks are first noted. The fact that the atypical head movements subside with increasing visual pursuit and fixation changing skill, lends further support to the idea that in many children OMA represents simply a delay in the maturation of normal saccadic and pursuit movements, and that the head swings are a compensation for the shortcoming. The frequently noted accompanying motor and language delays, suspected mental retardation and their gradual resolution, also suggest a maturational lag that is gradually overcome.

Why there should be a delay in gaining control of intentional eye movements is not clear, and ultimately raises the same questions as in connection with other assumed aetiologies; that is, what precisely is disrupted, how, and in what ways? Is OMA another case of a specific developmental delay, a concept used to explain apparently isolated slowness of maturation in other spheres of development? What is the significance of the so commonly reported co-occurrence of motor and language delay? Is this merely a result of the visual handicap, or does the triad represent a recognisable syndrome? Do the motor and language disruptions provide any clues as to the nature of the underlying defect in OMA, or, indeed, in more general types of praxic and higher mental developmental dysfunction? How far is OMA a true dyspraxia and how far is it only a case of simpler (that is, lower levels of control in the CNS) 'motor imbalance', lack of subcortical motor integration, or delay in establishing higher control over certain primitive reflexes?

Answers, even partial, to these questions await much more detailed knowledge of the mechanisms of normal voluntary eye control, the developmental stages in the acquisition of this control and the processes on which this all depends.

Acquired Ocular-motor Apraxia

Long before congenital OMA was described, reports had appeared of acquired disorders of voluntary eye movements. Cogan and Adams (1953) and De Renzi (1982) offer brief historical reviews. Terms applied to the disorder have included dyspraxia of gaze, gaze apraxia, gaze ataxia and ocular motor dyspraxia.

It shares with congenital OMA the impairment of volitional eye movements, both saccadic and pursuit, in the absence of external ocular muscle palsies, conjugate gaze paralysis or any other ophthalmoplegias. However, there are some important differences:

1. In acquired OMA, vertical and horizontal movements can be impaired (Monaco, Pirisi, Sechi and Cossu, 1980). Mills and Swanson (1978) recorded a case where voluntary vertical saccades only were involved, though it must be questioned whether their case description warrants the designation dyspraxia.

2. The characteristic head jerks of congenital OMA are absent in the acquired form. Instead, a common strategy used to gain refixation is to close the eyes, turn the head to face the new object of attention, then open the eyes again. This phenomenon is well described by the 19-year-old patient of Carecchi and Gainotti (1977). Other patients do not need to keep their eyes closed during the full excursion of the head, but manage with a slightly prolonged blink to detach their gaze from the object of attention.

3. There are two difficulties reported in conscious searching for an object. The first is an inability to defixate, with the eyes apparently locked on to their target. This spasm of fixation is widely described in the literature (De Renzi, 1982) and can be overcome by blinking, shutting the eyes or even introducing a blank screen before the eyes. The second is an inability to fixate a target at all. The person's eyes wander around aimlessly, even though they might be able to indicate gesturally or verbally where they should be looking. They may be able to maintain a fleeting fixation if they happen upon the target, but lose it just as soon again. It is unclear whether these represent two independent disabilities, or are complementary manifestations of a common underlying disordered mechanism. Denny-Brown's (1958) distinction between magnetic and repellent forces (p. 42) is worthwhile comparing in this context.

The woman described in Mills and Swanson (1978) had particular difficulties with mobility because of her spasm of fixation. She would fixate on an object in front of her while walking, which meant that as she approached it her eyes were drawn more and more into a downward gaze until she was actually looking at her feet and could no longer see where she was going. She could recentre her gaze by performing a vertical head thrust reminiscent of the horizontal thrust in congenital OMA. Unfortunately, the woman could not remember to use this strategy because of a co-existing memory problem, and would remain stuck in a downward gaze until someone reminded her what to do. This is the only acquired case reported with head thrusts.

4. Turning to all stimuli voluntarily is impaired in severe cases. Responses to auditory and tactile stimuli may be possible in milder cases. Therefore, these different conditions should be included in assessment.

5. Reflex activities are preserved as in congenital OMA. There may be two exceptions to this in acquired OMA: convergence on an object slowly moving towards the subject may be absent; and the blink reflex to a sudden threat may also be absent. Again, it is unclear whether these are part of the OMA disturbance, or are a result of commonly co-occurring deficits such as hemi-inattention, akinesia or simultanagnosia.

All other features are shared with congenital OMA. In milder cases, pursuit movements may be possible at slow velocities, but not at quicker ones. The OMA seldom occurs as an isolated disability. Typically, there are other problems, some secondary to the OMA, others due to other disruptions resulting from lesions in the same areas as those causing OMA.

Disabilities secondary to the OMA include reading, writing or any activities requiring scanning. Yarbus (1967) has demonstrated the handicap induced by ocular-motor disturbances in interpreting pictures or the features of complex objects. Tyler (1969), while not actually studying OMA patients, pointed to the correlation between poor language output and scanning deficits in dysphasics. It is interesting to speculate in this connection whether or not the presence of dysphasia may have impaired the directive function of language in the control of voluntary eye movements. Such a view would be in keeping with the work of Luria and Yudovitch (1956) and Luria (1973) as described on p. 136 in planning dyspraxia. Impaired scanning also leads to poor control of mobility: patients report that they are always tripping over or bumping into things. It will not always be immediately clear how far these difficulties are attributable to the OMA and how far they relate to commonly associated dysfunctions.

It may co-occur with all types of gestural and constructional dyspraxia. It may be found with frontal gait disturbance (see Chapter 6) (Cogan and Adams, 1952, case one); it may occur with planning dyspraxia and echopraxic behaviour (Monaco, Pirisi, Sechi *et al.*, 1980). Hypokinesia, (hemi-)inattention and visual field defects may be present. Various visual–spatial disorders can be found in some cases. These include topographical disorientation, visual agnosia, optic ataxia (p. 44), and misperception of size, depth and shape. Hécaen and De Ajuriaguerra (1954) include OMA as part of their definition of Balint's syndrome (see De Renzi, 1982; Hijdra and Meerwaldt, 1984), although Balint did not note it as a feature in his original case.

Localisation of the underlying pathology of acquired OMA remains problematical. A role in supranuclear ocular control has been claimed for many areas of the cortex. This is not surprising considering the phylogenetic and ontogenetic importance of vision to human behaviour — the capacity to react to sound and touch as well as sight, the co-ordination of eye movements with head and body movements, and the role in learning of vision, in association with sound and haptics. The schema arrived at by Holmes (1938) envisaged saccadic movements having a diffuse origin bilaterally in the frontal lobes, centred on Brodmann's area eight (see Figure 2.6a), while fixation and smooth pursuit were subserved by the occipital eye fields. Recent research, summarised by De Renzi (1982) and Hyvärinen (1982) does not fully bear out Holmes' hypotheses. This research points to a much more crucial role than hitherto assumed of the posterior parietal lobe, with Brodmann's area seven being the region of programming and initiation of ocular motor responses, particularly to visual stimuli with a definite location in space.

Whether or not acquired OMA represents a true dyspraxia, as defined in Chapter one, a release of more primitive reflexes, or some combination of explanations, awaits clarification of several matters. The precise nature of cortical and subcortical control over ocular movements needs to be established to ascertain which areas exert a truly planning influence and which areas are mediating or co-ordinating areas. It is probable that future investigation will disclose subtypes of OMA and permit a redefinition and classification of supranuclear disorders of ocular motion. Until then, while the difficulties encountered as described above are real enough, their inclusion within a dyspraxia scheme remains undecided.

Certain disorders of voluntary movement have been described and classified as types of dyspraxia whose status as true dyspraxias, in the sense discussed in Chapters 1 and 2, is disputed. The number of these goes far beyond those covered here (amnestic, bladder, eye-lid, palpebral . . .), which are chosen not just because the appreciation of their nature is important for the clinical necessities of recognition, assessment and rehabilitation. They are also chosen because understanding them adds further perspectives in comprehending the mechanisms and breakdown in the dyspraxias.

The callosal dyspraxias emphasise the importance of connecting pathways in the assembly and execution of motor programmes; they illustrate, *par excellence*, how certain dyspraxias can arise as a result of the disconnection of centres involved in praxis, rather than from damage to the centres themselves. This was recognised by Liepmann (1908) in his early formulations (see p. 9). The importance of overall cortical tone and maintenance of goal-directed behaviour is seen in frontal dyspraxia. Axial and gait dyspraxia are a reminder that higher cortical praxic functioning grows out of more global, less differentiated forms of action control (see Chapter 7). They also suggest that the classical divisions of cortical–subcortical, voluntary–automatic and pyramidal–extrapyramidal are not as strict as many texts would lead one to believe. The close relationship between perceptual, visual-spatial and motor components in action control is underlined in dressing dyspraxia.

Callosal Dyspraxia

Callosal lesions may come from surgical section (Gazzaniga, Bogen and Sperry, 1967; Bogen, 1969; Volpe, Siditis, Holtzman *et al.*, 1982) but, clinically, they are more likely to be seen after CVA (Barbizet, Degos, Duizabo *et al.*, 1974; Watson and Heilman, 1983), with neoplasms (Kretschmer, 1974), after head injury (Nakatani, Watanabe, Tashiro *et al.*, 1984), or in degenerative conditions (Barbizet, Degos, Lejeune *et al.*, 1978). There is variation in the symptomatic picture between the relatively pure lesions from surgical section and other causes. The latter give a less clear-cut picture because transcallosal disruption remains incomplete and because of the addition of symptoms associated with the involvement of intrahemispheric structures and pathways.

Figure 6.1: Medial View of Right Cerebral Hemisphere Showing Features of Corpus Callosum (Shaded): 1. Rostrum; 2. Anterior commissure; 3. Genu; 4. Trunk; 5. Cingulate gyrus; 6. Splenium

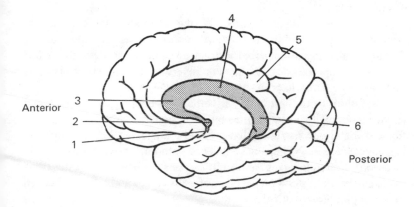

There is also longitudinal variation in the symptomatic picture (Gazzaniga *et al.*, 1967; Watson and Heilman, 1983). One can talk of (1) an acute stage; (2) a period after the immediate effects of surgical intervention or trauma have receded, during which interhemispheric disconnection difficulties are maximal; and (3) a period when relearning and reorganisation takes place through intrahemispheric changes, and the establishment or utilisation of subcortical interhemispheric routes.

The extent of improvement depends on all the usual factors (see Chapter 8). In surgical cases, the original reason (usually epilepsy) for intervention may influence outcome. The less damage caused by the original problem, the better the prognosis. The earlier the problem arises, the more likely there is to be bilateral representation of functions. This, and the extent to which intact fibres can take over or compensate for the role of damaged fibres in incomplete disconnection, may influence the symptomatic picture.

Dyspraxia is only one of many sequelae of callosal disruption. There are two main types (in a right-handed person without mixed laterality): a unilateral left ideomotor and a unilateral right constructional dyspraxia.

Unilateral Left Ideomotor Dyspraxia

Using the normal procedure for assessing ideomotor dyspraxia (Chapter 2), callosal involvement might be suspected if there is:
1. Faultless right hand performance to verbal instruction.
2. A marked difference in the left hand between poor performance to verbal command, relatively good response to imitation and normal use of real objects.

Thus, despite being unable to raise the left middle finger to verbal command, a patient will succeed when *shown* what is expected; or, despite an inability after verbal instruction to demonstrate with the left hand how to open a door, the patient nevertheless may easily open the door with the same hand when they leave the room.

The failure of the left hand on verbal instructions can even extend to when pointing to objects named by the examiner. Barbizet *et al.* (1978) found this feature so striking that they even suggested the label 'aphasic apraxia'. Some individuals may succeed with left-hand pointing if only one-word directions are given, or if the vital information in the command can be understood on the basis of a key word, and is not embedded in a complex grammatical structure.

Another feature that may be found, especially in the early stages of recovery, is a contrast between left limb performance for proximally (swinging the leg; saluting) and distally (adopting various finger postures) controlled movements to verbal command.

The reasons for this dyspraxic picture are: the poor language capacity of the right hemisphere; and the poor ipsilateral motor control exercised by the left hemisphere. The success of some people on single object pointing rests with the ability of the right hemisphere to understand single words. The better performance on proximally controlled movements derives from the better ipsilateral innervation of this musculature.

Performance standards gradually rise over a period of months, with gross distal movement (opening and closing the fist) preceding finer control. The dyspraxia may not be immediately apparent in everyday activities where recovery is good, but it may be demonstrable on specific testing or when the person is fatigued, tense or presented with novel tasks even up to years later (Zaidel and Sperry, 1977).

Left Unilateral Dysgraphia

This disorder accompanies the dyspraxia. Block capitals may be copied adequately without appreciation of their literal value. Transcribing from cursive to capital script or vice versa is not possible. The patient may not be able to copy what he has just produced using his right hand —

see Barbizet *et al.* (1978) for an example. In keeping with the rudimentary language capacity of the right hemisphere, single and overlearned (name, numbers) words may be written with the left hand, but phrases and sentences are impossible. Occasionally, where relatively good ipsilateral control has been established, patients may proceed beyond the one word level, particularly if they have learned to capitalise on the better use of proximal musculature (see page 214 for exploitation of this in hemiplegics).

Watson and Heilman's (1983) patient had an apraxic dysgraphia in the left hand with normal right-handed writing. However, she was able to type grammatically well-formed sentences with her left hand, since she had a CVA that spared the posterior callosum. Sugishita, Toyokura, Yoshioka *et al.* (1980) described a patient with section of the posterior part of the splenium, who had no dyspraxia of the left hand but did have a dysphasic dyspraxia. Gersh and Damasio (1981) reported a similar case. Compare also Brown *et al.* (1983).

Apart from variations in the symptomatic picture according to the site of lesion that are demonstrated by these cases, they also have important implications for the understanding of motor programming processes. Further discussion of this is found in the works cited.

Unilateral Right Constructional Dyspraxia

While the left hand displays ideomotor dyspraxia to verbal command, the right hand is constructionally dyspraxic, being unable to execute visual–spatial tasks such as copying geometric figures, stick design tests, or spontaneous drawing. Productions are limited to scrawls, spatially disrupted attempts or slavish copying of one detail after another. Bogen (1969) borrowed the term 'dyscopia' to denote the inability to copy shapes.

However, the right hand is able to write normally, though in some cases there may be some spatial disturbance to the layout of letters and words. Poor right-handed copying ability is in contrast to good left-handed copying.

A further detectable dissociation is the improvement in construction by the right hand under verbal guidance, while the left hand is unable to produce shapes under purely verbal direction, despite effortless ability in copying the same (Bogen, 1969; Barbizet *et al.*, 1978). The phenomenon of intermanual conflict (see below) is often encountered where constructional tasks are attempted using both hands — the right hand tends to disorganise the ordered structure produced by the left hand.

Associated Features

In addition to the dyspraxic manifestations, there are several well recognised features of manual behaviour and co-ordination that may accompany the dyspraxia, which are also attributable to the interhemispheric disconnection. Many of these signs and symptoms may lead to the diagnosis of mental or psychiatric disorder, but it is stressed here that, in callosal lesions, they are direct functional manifestations of the disconnection.

One common phenomenon is dissociation between whole body movements (getting up; turning) and the actions carried out by the hands. There may also be a mismatch between what the person is saying (left hemisphere dominant) and what the left hand is doing (right hemisphere dominant). Such non-congruity can also be observed between facial expression and verbal content. However, the variability of this in the normal population, let alone among brain-damaged people, renders it unreliable as a useful sign of hemispheric disconnection.

Intermanual Conflict. This arises from the dissociation between the actions of two limbs when bimanual co-ordination is required. Akelaitis (1944–45) labelled this 'diagnostic dyspraxia'. One of his patients would open a drawer or door with his right hand and the left hand would close it immediately. Barbizet *et al.*'s (1978) patient was given the verbal instruction to wrap up two books in a piece of paper that was slightly too small. The left hand, unconscious of the verbal instruction, read the visual clues that suggested he remove one book to enable the paper to reach round at least one book. However, the right hand kept putting it back, in keeping with the verbal instruction. More embarrassing for the patient, while out shopping, he several times accepted the purchase with his right hand but at the same time the left hand took back the money he had just laid down on the counter. The woman described by Watson *et al.* (1983) one day went to her wardrobe to select a blouse to wear. Independently, her left hand chose one, her right hand another; she put the left arm in one, her right in the other. Then the left arm pulled the right blouse off, only for it to be put back on again by the right hand. The on-off struggle continued until her daugher intervened.

Alien Hand. Even if bimanual co-operation is not necessary, the left hand may still act in an unpredictable and seemingly uncontrollable fashion. Brion and Jedynak (1972) called this the foreign, or alien hand sign. Barbizet *et al.*'s (1978) patient asked his wife to get his cigarettes out of his left pocket, because he felt he could not get his hand to do it.

But as his wife went to do it, his left hand took the cigarettes out of the pocket, put them on the table, and then put them back in his pocket. At other times, the left hand might assume 'strange' postures or carry out other actions seemingly (for the patient and the onlooker) out of the blue.

The surprise of sufferers when their alien hand behaves outside of their conscious control has been accepted as another feature of inter-hemispheric disconnection by Brion and Jedynak (1975), who labelled it 'interhemispheric autocriticism'. These happenings occur as chronic symptoms of commissural disruption.

These phenomena can be evaluated by careful observation or careful questioning when the report is taken. Certain tasks may elicit the behaviour in the clinical context. Naturalistic tasks like the book wrapping exercise of Barbizet *et al.* (1978), or any undertaking that will require a high degree of intermanual co-operation — especially ones unfamiliar to the patient — are suitable. For instance, the person succeeds when instructed to tap a regular rhythm with either hand singly. Instructed to tap the rhythm simultaneously with both hands, he may succeed at slow rates but completely lose it on speeding up. Tapping alternatively with one hand and then the other is impossible. Usually, the left hand simply ceases tapping while the right taps on alone.

Pseudo-Neglect. The feeling of many 'split-brain' patients that they have little control over their left limbs may lead to a pseudo-neglect or under use, in as far as they do not attempt acts with it, sensing failure will result (for example, the man described by Barbizet *et al.* whose cigar-ettes were in his left pocket). The left-sided neglect may further derive from reduced dominant hemisphere control.

Impaired Sensory Transfer. The person is unable to replicate finger postures from one hand to the other without visual feedback. Neither can he indicate on, or with, the opposite limb the place in which he has been touched contralaterally. By the same token, patients cannot retrieve an object matching one held concealed in the contralateral hand.

Left Tactile Anomia. A further consequence of the loss of inter-hemispheric transfer of information is the inability of the person to name an object in the left hand by touch alone. This may result from astereognosis where lesions extend into the right hemisphere. This cause of failure can be excluded in two ways:
1. One can observe whether the person can manipulate and use the object

appropriately, despite not being able to name it;
2. The person can be encouraged to choose, with the same hand, a matching object from a selection inside a bag or covered box.

There are other behavioural features that can be demonstrated, but they have only peripheral relevance to praxis and so are not detailed here. These include hemialexia, double hemianopia, unilateral 'verbal' anosmia and spatial dyscalculia. A discussion of these can be found in Bogen (1985). Variations in the above picture can be observed in cases of incomplete destruction of transcallosal fibres.

Incomplete Disconnection

Volpe *et al.* (1982) studied people who had undergone only partial section of the callosum, or complete section in stages. Among their conclusions, they confirmed that each hemisphere, under the correct stimulus conditions, had the potential for contralateral distal control. In particular, the right hemisphere may contribute uniquely to some visual-motor tasks. This has direct relevance to developing possible compensatory strategies in rehabilitation (see Chapter 8).

Volpe *et al.* established that: posterior sectioning is sufficient to disrupt acts requiring interhemispheric integration; posterior section is sufficient to produce functional disconnection of distal muscles; and interhemispheric transfer of non-verbal sensorimotor information depends on specific posterior fibres; an isolated mid-callosal lesion is enough to affect tactile transfer; the anterior trunk and/or genu does not transfer critical visual or sensorimotor information for distal control, and neither is it able to transfer visual images that elicit motor activity, nor the specific motor programme needed to carry out the appropriate movement.

Watson and Heilman (1983) described a woman who suffered a CVA at the junction of the genu and body of the corpus callosum, sparing the posterior sections. There was no direct cortical involvement. In the acute stage there was functionally complete disconnection due to associated oedema. At this time, her left hand showed an ideational dyspraxia to verbal command, while the right hand managed normally. At about three weeks post-onset, her left hand demonstrated a mixed ideational–ideomotor dyspraxia. With functional recovery of the posterior callosum, she had return of left-hand tactile naming ability, and the earlier hemialexia resolved. By seven weeks post-onset she had a left hand dysgraphia and ideomotor dyspraxia. There was proximal–distal differentiation in accuracy of execution. Despite the dysgraphia, she could type syntactically well-formed sentences with her left hand. There was a right-hand constructional dyspraxia, and she suffered from the alien hand sign.

Neighbourhood Signs and Symptoms

Testing for or recognising hemisphere disconnection symptoms may be clouded by lateralising effects if lesions encroach on intrahemispheric pathways or structures. Extension into the left hemisphere may produce dysphasia and true dyspraxias of the right hand, and the latter may be masked by a hemiparesis. There may be a unilateral leg weakness or paralysis in CVA of the anterior cerebral artery.

Involvement of the left prefrontal cortex may result in akinetic mutism, with the mutism persisting beyond the mute phase reported as typical immediately succeeding acute disconnection (Watson and Heilman, 1983; Bogen, 1985). Prefrontal involvement may also lead to behaviour and personality shifts, both of which add to the picture of non-typical behaviour secondary to the disconnections, rendering reliable assessment difficult, and lessening the chances of the sufferer being able to benefit from spontaneous re-organisation and rehabilitative intervention. Frontal trauma may also be associated with gait problems, forced grasping, groping reflex, motor impersistence, perseveration and ocular motor disorders, all of which are absent in purely callosal lesions.

Extension of lesions into the right hemisphere may produce a true constructional dyspraxia in the left hand as well as spatial dysgraphia (page 81), in addition to the language-based dysgraphia due to disconnection from the language hemisphere. Common right hemisphere lesion sequelae are also likely in such cases — hemi-inattention/neglect, visual–spatial disturbances and denial.

Compression or invasion of midbrain and brain stem structures will give rise to additional pyramidal and extrapyramidal features — spasticity, ataxia, hyper-, hypokinesia. These may be manifested as speech (dysarthric) gait and co-ordination difficulties, beyond the disco-ordination due to disconnection. Kretschmer (1974) has described the associated clinical findings caused by the spread of neoplasms beyond the corpus callosum proper.

The above details are those found in right-handers with no significant indication of shared or reversed dominance. Findings among left-handers are seldom the exact reversal of dextrals, and the picture is further complicated in cases of non-absolute dominance or anomalous dextrality (that is, right-handedness with right hemisphere dominance). Readers are referred to the specialist works cited for discussion of these matters.

Frontal Dyspraxia

It is impossible to set out in this brief context the complexities and challenges associated with the neuropsychological study of the frontal lobes in their normal — let alone abnormal — state. Readers are referred for this to works such as Luria (1973), Hécaen and Albert (1978), Jouandet and Gazzaniga (1979) and Damasio (1985). A short account is offered here of the type of disruption to action found in prefrontal lesions.

The main behaviours associated with the frontal lobe syndromes that impinge on motor performance are: a tendency to inattentiveness and distractibility with an inability to attend selectively to a task, and increased orientation to non-relevant stimuli; perseveration of part actions and strategies leading to inertia of response; and depressed perceptual and other problem-solving behaviour from defective scanning and impairment in the analysis of complex objects and situations. Affective disorders, disinterest and inactivity, may be part of the picture in some patients, while memory problems, dysphasia, other dyspraxias and hemiparesis add to the complex of symptoms in others.

Several authors (Luria, 1973; Roy, 1978; Truelle, Fardoun, Delestre *et al.*, 1979) have spoken of a frontal or primary planning dyspraxia. Here, individual actions that require only a simple, immediate response ('Open your mouth'; 'Raise your arm'; 'Pick up the glass in front of you') are fluently performed. Breakdown occurs when the execution and solution of an action requires insight into the problem (for example, how to open a tin of peas); the planning of a complex motor response that goes beyond the immediate context and will involve both adjustment of personal space and manipulation in external space; correct sequencing of sub-parts of the act; and running of the 'programme' until its completion.

In frontal dyspraxia, the ability to organise an overall action and regulate and monitor its execution are impaired. This is not a dyspraxia in the strictest sense, as it can be seen to be part of a more general cognitive, organisational dysfunction unrestricted to motor behaviour. However, it gives rise to characteristic errors that can be seen on observation or elicited in specific tests.

In severe cases, the person is unable to begin the action, even though they have all the necessary utensils and can repeat the instruction. They will sit there, look puzzlingly at the objects and declare that they do not know what to do with them. In less severe cases they may make a correct first move, but fail to carry the action through.

Figure 6.2: Drawing of a Bicycle By a Patient With an Anterior Communicating Artery Aneurysm

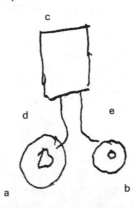

In Figure 6.2 the patient, who had an anterior communicating artery aneurysm, was asked to draw a bike. She held the pencil over the paper for a minute or so and then said she did not know how to. It was suggested that she start with the wheels: she drew the outer ring of (a). She was asked where the other wheel was, and drew the inner circle. The patient was told to put the back wheel behind the front: she drew the two circles of (b) but, after further deliberation, said she still did not know what to do. The frame was mentioned, and (c) was produced. When told to fix the frame and wheels together she drew (d) and then (e). She was well aware it bore no resemblance to a bike.

More characteristically, patients start the action but it is easily derailed. Stimuli intrude from the outside, or innerward associations send the contents of their activity off at a tangent. Thus, goal-directed behaviour is replaced by a series of isolated movements that bear less and less resemblance to the original intention. This happens despite the person demonstrating that they have retained the instruction.

Getting dressed in the morning, such a patient may start off correctly, then, seeing the toothbrush, break off dressing to clean their teeth. Having done that, they may notice their night clothes on the bed, decide to pull them on over the clothes they already have on, and get back into bed. Making a cup of tea, they may suddenly notice the sink and washing-up liquid and proceed to put the cup and saucer, sugar, teapot and tea into the bowl for washing up. One should recall the utilisation behaviour of Lhermitte (1983) on page 43.

Figure 6.3 gives another example of this type of derailment. The woman concerned was trying to *write* 'wee girl' to describe the cookie-

Figure 0.3: Drawing By a Patient Trying to Write 'Wee Girl'

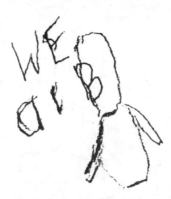

jar picture in the Boston Aphasia Examination (Goodglass and Kaplan, 1983). She started *writing*, but being 'distracted' by the picture changed to *drawing* a wee girl.

On testing imitation of gestures the frontal dyspraxic performs well on isolated items. However, if the examiner carries out a competing action (for example, raising an arm to indicate when the patient is to put their hand behind their back), then the patient's response is easily deflected and they tend to give an echopraxic reply, imitating the examiner. Instructions such as 'Lift your right hand when I lift my left', or 'Turn round when I sit down', are virtually impossible — even when comprehension of the task is confirmed.

The same distractibility can be seen in conversation. The person is easily led astray by other talk going on in the environment; this may be despite the clinician's frustrated attempts to get the patient to answer direct questions. At another time, the clinician might have tried in vain to get the person to look at an object or to follow a finger while testing vision or eye movements, yet in the middle of all this they may suddenly fixate on a stain on their pullover, or follow the nurse with their eyes as she walks down the ward.

Other derailments involve more complex or unfamiliar actions being distracted by or resolving into more elementary or habitual responses. One woman who had worked in a greengrocer's shop was given an orange to eat by the woman in the next hospital bed. Immediately, she got up to find a paper bag to put it in and gave it back to her. Having said goodbye to a patient, she followed the author up the ward. Asked where she was going, she replied, 'To see you out of the door', even though she knew she was in hospital.

Figure 6.4: Drawing of a Cat, Without a Model. The patient knew it was unsuccessful, but was unable to proceed

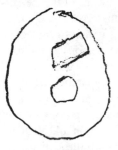

Figure 6.5: Drawing of a Flower, Without a Model (Produced After the Attempt at Figure 6.3)

Figure 6.6: Copy of the Flower, Produced Immediately After Figure 6.4

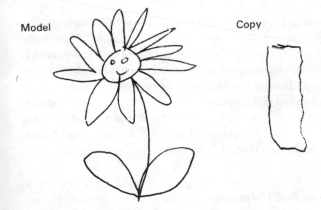

Model   Copy

Perseveration is also a feature of frontal dyspraxia. This is not only of single part-actions (for example, writing TABLE as TTT or TAAA), but can involve perseveration of strategies used to solve problems, or perceptual features in drawing. The reader should notice, apart from the dissolution of the spatial aspects, the perseveration both of the rectangular shape and the inclusion of this inside a closed form in the Figures 6.4, 6.5 and 6.6.

Typically, the person is aware of their errors, even though they are unable to say why or how the error came about. However, they are incapable of utilising the information to correct their actions. This occurs even in instances where the person is able to remember and verbalise precisely what they are meant to do.

Frontal dyspraxia can be seen to be part of a more general breakdown in the planning and regulation of goal-oriented behaviour. It may also be associated with other manifestations of prefrontal dysfunction.

There may be poverty of action and verbalisation, ranging from the aspontaneity of akinetic mutism through various degrees of lack of initiative, slowness in initiation, inability to sustain simple repetitive or complex movements, and disinclination to act. Left to themselves, frontal dyspraxic patients may neglect (rather than actually forget) to get up and do not wash or dress, or do so only partially. Daily living activities are done without apparent care or interest. They do not seek out personal contact and fail to join in with groups unless constantly prompted.

Aspontaneity or neglect may be restricted to one side: they may succeed when requested to lift each arm individually but when asked to raise both together, one arm is left down, or lifted but soon falls. When tapping a regular rhythm with both feet or hands, the aspontaneous side soon stops or never starts.

There is insufficient space here to discuss all the features that, ideally, should be considered in frontal dyspraxia. These include the presence of other dyspraxia types and symptoms of interhemispheric disconnection. It entails possible hemispheric differences, and the symptomatology of bifrontal lesions. Subcortical extension of involvement also adds to the picture (see axial and gait dyspraxia, the next sections in this chapter). Likewise, changes in effect may contribute to the frontal syndrome. These factors are discussed in the works cited (Luria, 1973; Hécaen and Albert, 1978, Jouandet and Gazzaniga, 1979).

Axial Movements and Dyspraxia

One sees patients who are unable to turn over in bed; sit up from the lying position, or from a chair; co-ordinate limb and whole body movements in carrying out actions such as bowing, curtseying or turning round to sit down in a chair; and who have difficulty achieving correct posture when standing or sitting. These disabilities occur in instances where deficits in power, tone, co-ordination and sensation are absent, or insufficient to wholly account for the behaviour. The label 'dyspraxia' has been applied to these difficulties by some workers. However, clinicians differ about which behaviours are designated as representing the dyspraxia. Others dispute whether dyspraxia is the cause at all.

Lakke, in a series of studies (Lakke, r.d. Burg and Wiegman, 1982; Lakke, Van Weerden and Staal-Schreinemachers, 1984) noted that pharmacological therapy in parkinsonism affected only the classical symptoms of tremor, rigidity and akinesia. It did not alleviate dysfunction in certain learned, voluntarily initiated, 'automatic' movements like standing up, or turning round. When turning over in bed, these patients often adopt abnormal strategies, such as levering the arm against the bed, markedly bending at the knees before the turn, or initiating the turn with the pelvis or legs. This contrasts with normal turning while asleep, under severe emotional pressure or in time to music. In view of the variability of performance and the presence of the dysfunction with otherwise able motor performance, Lakke *et al.* labelled this phenomenon 'axial dyspraxia'.

Denny-Brown (1958) described many similar behaviours under his concept of magnetic and repellent dyspraxia (see page 42) in which not only axial and postural movement is disordered, but also limb and facial movements.

Poeck, Lehmkuhl and Willmes (1982) described a different set of behaviours under the title 'axial dyspraxia'. They reported ideomotor-type errors on tasks involving head and eye movements, and commands to take one step forwards or back, or to lift both shoulders. Poeck *et al.* also pointed out that many of the items for oral dyspraxia assessment (cough, wiggle nose, non-vegetative breathing) are axial, midline actions.

On the other hand, Geschwind (1965) remarked on the striking preservation of axial whole-body movements in patients with definite limb dyspraxia. Indeed, one finds patients who fail relatively simple items from the ideomotor test battery to verbal and gestural command, and yet flawlessly perform instructions to 'stand up and turn around', or 'go to the window and bow'. The disparity is often a source of disagreement between health care workers and relatives concerning the severity of dyspraxia and dysphasia.

Geschwind hypothesised that whole-body movements are spared because they utilise different anatomical arrangements to the limbs (see Freund and Hummelsheim, 1984, for support for this in humans). Roeltgen and Heilman (1983) conjectured that comprehension of certain subsets of speech may be represented separately from other subsets and therefore, are spared when other comprehension is impaired.

Alternatively, or as well, comprehension for whole-body movements and their engrams may reside in the non-dominant hemisphere or be bilaterally represented.

The explanations for hemiplegic writing offered by Brown, Leader and Blum (1983) also have relevance here. They believe that the destruction of a surface, asymmetric cortical (page 161) 'level' in the linguistic and praxic microgenetic process results in action planning terminating at a less differentiated stage. This older (phylo- and ontogenetically) motor planning system subserving axial and proximal movements is normally submerged below the more recent distal, differentiated control. Nevertheless, dissolution of the latter can spare the former, which then becomes accessible and the new endpoint of action elaboration.

These groups (Denny-Brown, 1958; Geschwind, 1965; Poeck *et al.*, 1982; Lakke *et al.*, 1984) are obviously talking about different things. Poeck *et al.* talk of midline movements, and in concentrating on head — and especially eye — movements, are assessing actions well removed from the postural and whole-body control that is the central attention of others.

Denny-Brown is discussing primarily abnormal reflex activity. Other than saying that this type of behaviour does occur (page 41 to 42), and complicates the management of patients, it does not have an immediate place in the consideration of praxis, and so will not be covered in any more detail here.

Lakke *et al.* are not discussing a dyspraxia in the traditional sense of the word: to say that the disability occurs with normal tone, power and sensation, and that the actions are possible in *other* contexts is not sufficient. Dyspraxia is characterised by variation of performance in the same context, as well as across situations. It is also characterised by specific types of derailment, and not simply by non-initiation.

However, as a disorder of the voluntary initiation of automatic acts, the axial dyspraxia of Lakke *et al.* represents a disorder at the junction between subcortical, automatic, primitive postural processes and volitional activity. Whitaker (1983) has argued that the automatic-voluntary divide represents less mutually exclusive poles than two ends of a continuum. Such a continuum is also implicit in the work of Piaget (1936/77) and Brown (1977).

The argument for seeing a continuity between automatic and volitional is taken up again in the next section. As regards axial movements and dyspraxia, all the views outlined above are accurate and not necessarily conflicting. There are disorders of axial movement close to other dyspraxias, but it is maintained here that it is inaccurate to speak of axial dyspraxia as a separate entity in the way that one speaks of ideomotor and ideational dyspraxia.

Gait Dyspraxia

This is the label given by some to a characteristic disturbance of gait associated particularly with prefrontal lesions. There is relative agreement concerning its description, but its classification as a dyspraxia is disputed.

Clinical Description

The disorder is manifested, of course, most clearly when the person is asked to walk. In severe cases (provided the person can stand), on trying to walk forwards, it seems as if the patient's feet are glued to the floor. Despite much apparent effort, he is unable to lift his foot from the ground, or move it along, and he may declare that he has forgotten how to walk. In less severe instances, initiation of movement may be hesitant, followed by a shuffling 'slipping-clutch' gait (Denny-Brown, 1958). Excursions of the leg are small. Some people may step out with one foot and then try to make the next step with the same foot, or lift the foot without advancing it. If obstacles, or even just lines on the floor, are placed in their path, they are unable to step over them. Stairs are out of the question. Turning is impossible or achieved only after much manoeuvring and effort. The tendency to fall is ever present.

Not only is the person unable to propel their body forwards, but they are also impaired in carrying out other tasks. They are unable to stand on one leg; they cannot pretend to kick a ball, stub out a cigarette or trace figures or letters on the floor with their foot. Reports have appeared of patients being assisted by the presence of a real ball or cigarette (Meyer and Barron, 1960), but this has not been experienced in personal cases. Typically, the arms hang motionless when some locomotion is possible, and the face is expressionless. The head may be held in an abnormal attitude and overall posture may be distorted (Knutsson and Lying-Tunell, 1985).

These problems while standing are in contrast to performance when the legs are not weight-bearing, for example, while lying, sitting or being supported so that the patient can stand on one leg. Sufferers can then faultlessly pretend how to kick a ball, pedal a bike, trace shapes or tap their foot, which they were unable to do minutes before while standing ordinarily. However, certain more complex movements, especially if both legs must be co-ordinated, remain defective or impossible.

Figure 6.7: Gait Dyspraxic Patient in Supine Position Attempting to Rise

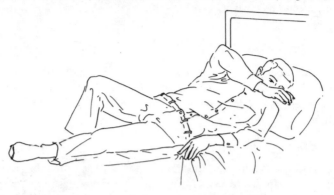

Figure 6.8: The Same Patient Attempting to Rise by Pulling on the Bed Head

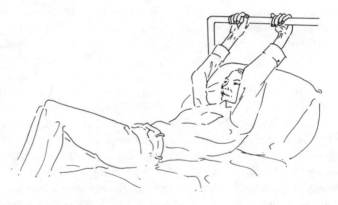

However, problems go beyond those of gait. Rising from supine, the person struggles and may succeed only in raising the head or turning on their side (Figure 6.7). Sufferers may try to pull themselves up on the cot sides (Figure 6.8). Sitting up may be difficult even with assistance. Once sitting, such patients experience problems swinging their legs over the side of the bed. They may not be able to stand if already seated, appearing to be glued to the chair (Figure 6.9) or they finish up in general extension. They are not able to bend over if standing. Thus, disruption of axial or whole-body movements can also be seen to be a feature of gait dyspraxia.

Upper limb involvement is not uncommon and typically shows the grasp reactions described on page 41, with consequent disruption of manual activities. Eye movement can be affected with slowed smooth

Figure 6.9: Gait Dyspraxic Patient 'Glued' to Chair, and Unable to Rise

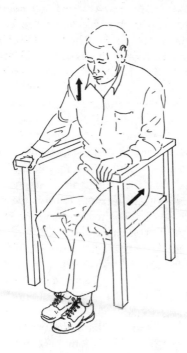

pursuit, or pursuit only by a succession of saccades. Pointing with the impaired limbs is dysmetric, but it is not a rhythmical, swaying misreaching as in cerebellar ataxia. Reaching performance may be improved by increased attention and practice. A fine, rapid tremor appearing in action is also commonly reported. This, too, contrasts with the slow, coarse tremor of ataxia.

There is no weakness or sensory loss on neurological examination. If there is, it is insufficient to account for the difficulties. Grasp reflexes are usually present not only in the feet but also in the hands, and a sucking reflex may be elicited. Passive manipulation of the limbs commonly provokes counterholding, or *Gegenhalten*, whereby there is increased resistance as if the person is trying to push the examiner away.

Cases have been reported in the literature by Sandyk (1983); Estañol (1981); Deodato, Di Rosa, Meduri *et al.* (1979) and Knutsson and Lying-Tunell (1985). Meyer and Barron (1960) made a thorough review of studies and views of gait dyspraxia since its conception in the nineteenth century as well as presenting seven patients of their own.

Denny-Brown (1958) described the same phenomenon under the label 'magnetic dyspraxia'. He also covered the contrasting disorder of repellent dyspraxia supposedly due to unchecked avoiding reactions released after parietal lobe lesion. The hand and arm characteristics of this have been mentioned above (pages 41 and 42). The tendency in walking in so-called repellent dyspraxia, as with upper limb actions, is to withdraw from any contact, but if contact is made it is light and fleeting. Gait is performed with overextended toes, flexed knees and with the feet lifted high off the ground, though Denny-Brown notes that gait may be shuffling in bilateral lesions, and the overextended toes predispose to falling backwards. It is not only sitting up that may pose problems. Turning round from standing to sit in a seat may be difficult also. The patient may make several tentative but abortive approaches (see also axial movements, pages 140–2). In trying to draw the chair up to the table, they may succeed only in pushing it around the room, being unable to lift it because of the repellent postures.

The cases of gait dyspraxia as discussed in the above references all involve some kind of frontal lesion. These include neoplasm, vascular aetiologies (Meyer and Barron, 1960), communicating hydrocephalus (Estañol, 1981; Knutsson and Lying-Tunell, 1985), cerebral and basal ganglia calcifications (Sandyk, 1983), and generalised atrophy more marked in the right posterior medial frontal region (Deodato *et al.*, 1979). Lesions and limb involvement are both bilateral and unilateral; clouding of consciousness and impaired mentation are frequent co-findings. Psychosocial, language, memory and affective disorders may also be present, in keeping with frontal lobe pathology. The associated features improve where lesions are reversible, as does the gait disorder.

Differential Diagnosis

The disorder usually considered liable to be confused with gait dyspraxia is cerebellar ataxia. Indeed, some writers (see Meyer and Barron, 1960) have discussed gait dyspraxia under the label 'frontal ataxia', though others maintain that the latter is a separate disturbance.

Meyer and Barron list among the distinguishing features the fast non-shuffling gait of the cerebellar ataxic, with the feet being lifted easily from the ground, compared to the slow, short step, shuffling progression of the dyspraxic. Hesitant initiation and poverty of movement characterise the dyspraxic, while ready initiation is seen in the ataxic. Execution of real or pantomimed acts is clumsily but rapidly carried out by ataxics, while only hesitantly and slowly, if at all, by gait dyspraxics. The latter are able to perform ably in a supine position what they cannot do when standing; for ataxics, performance is essentially the same in both positions. According to Meyer and Barron (1960), the gait dyspraxic improves when walking on all fours, while the ataxic remains as impaired as when upright. Resistance to passive movement is decreased in ataxics but increased in gait dyspraxia, usually developing into rigidity.

Associated signs and symptoms are different in the frontal syndrome. Grasp reflexes, perseveration, disorders of mentation, memory and affect are absent in lesions restricted to the cerebellum. Cerebellar involvement may involve scanning-type dysarthric speech, while akinetic mutism, transcortical motor (adynamic) dysphasia or Broca's dysphasia will more likely accompany frontal lesions.

In trying to resolve the confusion over gait dyspraxia and frontal ataxia, Meyer and Barron proposed three types of (pre)frontal gait disturbance:
1. Ataxic gait may result from large space-occupying lesions displacing intracranial structures and causing cerebello-medullary compression;
2. Expanding lesions might also result in interference from displacement and compression of the eighth cranial nerve. This would bring about labyrinthine vertigo and ataxia;
3. Localised frontal damage, not causing displacement, would not cause ataxia, but would result in what Meyer and Barron have termed 'gait dyspraxia'.

The notion of frontal ataxia, however, remains unclear.

Is Dyspraxia of Gait a Dyspraxia?

Meyer and Barron (1960) offer as their definition and justification for inclusion under a dyspraxia label the fact that there is 'loss of ability to properly use the lower limbs in the act of walking which cannot be accounted for by demonstrable sensory impairment or motor weakness' (p. 279). However, the mere absence of these features is insufficient to warrant classification as a dyspraxia.

To be a dyspraxia, there must also be errors of inclusion and not just exclusion. For example, performance should not be just clumsy or absent, but should show substitutions or distortions of actions. Execution should be correct on occasions, and impaired at other times. Differences between erect and supine performance would not fulfil this criterion. Kerschensteiner *et al.* (1975) also rightly point out the conceptual misthinking in assuming that there can be a dyspraxia of a single function — here gait. One does not speak of waving-goodbye dyspraxia of the upper limbs or smiling dyspraxia of the face.

Kerschensteiner *et al.* (1975) hypothesise that a lesion to the parasagittal motor association cortex might produce gait dyspraxia, but one would expect there to be dyspraxic errors for other leg actions, and not just walking. However, lesions here would also cause initiation problems, counterholding and grasp reflexes, thus rendering it difficult to isolate a pure dyspraxic element. Poeck *et al.* (1982), who demonstrated dyspraxia in the lower limbs, did not find that it caused these gait problems.

That gait dyspraxia is a misnomer is already implicit in the analyses of Meyer and Barron (1960), and others. Lower limb function is not the only action involved; truncal, arm, hand and oral movements are also a part. Walking is impaired, and so too are other foot and leg movements, as well as sitting up, turning over and writing.

As correctly noted by Denny-Brown (1958), the disorder is better explained by the interference to normal movement by abnormal reflex activity. Performance is improved by inhibition of these reflexes, which is not true for genuine dyspraxias: these are disruptions at a higher level of organisation.

However, gait dyspraxia, or frontal gait disturbance as Geschwind (1965) prefers to call it, is not fully accounted for by the abnormal reflex explanation. Certain features suggest that a clearer understanding is to be sought in other directions, which would place the disorder at the interface between automatic and volitional behaviour. In the literature, gait dyspraxia has been contrasted with ataxia, but comparison with hypokinetic movement disorders appears to be more appropriate.

It shares with parkinsonism the hesitancy and slowness of initiation, the expressionless face, the immobile arms and the tendency to festination, and sudden arrest or freezing of movement. Reports of freezing in abnormal postures and general aspontaneity link it with catatonia and akinetic mutism. Impairment of bimanual or bipedal co-ordination and the complete inability to carry out complex sequential tasks are also shared features with parkinsonism (Stern, Mayeux, Rosen *et al.*, 1983) and frontal planning disorders (Luria, 1973; Roy, 1978; p. 136).

Considering the richness of interconnections between basal ganglia and frontal and prefrontal cortex, it is not surprising that lesions of these areas should give similar clinical pictures. Much recent work has pointed to basal ganglia functions far beyond the traditional role ascribed to them of balancing muscle tone between agonists and antagonists. This suggests also a role in activating and modulating higher cortical function.

Evarts and Wise (1984) cite evidence supporting the idea that basal ganglia and frontal association cortex work as an integrated system for the preparation of complex movements, and that they are essential for self-initiated, self-guided and spontaneous actions. (It is interesting to note in this connection the improvement in gait seen with external guided support, for example, feet painted on the floor, metronome and so on.)

Thus motor symptomatology in basal ganglia and frontal lobe disruption may be understood partly in relation to disruption to this system. Marsden (1984) has reviewed work indicating that in parkinsonism difficulty exists in the automatic execution of learnt motor plans, which themselves may be formulated in premotor and other frontal areas. Further, parkinsonians have difficulty in switching from one programme to another and specifying (in terms of ballistic control) the detailed accuracy of these actions.

The intermittent light photography and electromyographic recordings made by Knutsson and Lying-Tunell (1985) in normal-pressure hydrocephalus gait dyspraxics, demonstrated disruption to the normal phasic activation of anti-gravity muscles over the hip and knee joints. This correlated with the 'glued' stance and slow, small angular displacements when walking. Again, commonalities with parkinsonian abnormalities are apparent.

Gait is a learned motor activity normally executed under automatic, subconscious control. It requires bilateral co-ordination and careful regulation of force and range of movements in maintaining balance, direction and changes of speed and direction. These features and functions are impaired in gait dyspraxia. While this does not represent a disorder of action in the sense discussed elsewhere in this book, it is a breakdown of voluntary control, complicated by other disruptions (reflex) to motor performance. It is suggested that a greater understanding of its nature and underlying pathology will be gained by examining it in the context of the assembly and generation of skilled movement, and the automatic execution of learnt motor plans.

Dressing Dyspraxia

Clinicians have long recognised patients who fail to dress properly despite adequate power, sensation, balance, attention and understanding of the task. Where any of these deficits has been present, they have been insufficient to account either for the degree of impairment or the nature of the errors experienced.

Clinical Description

In marked cases, sufferers are unable to even start dressing themselves. They pick up garments, look puzzlingly at them, twist and turn them, put them down to try another item, ask what to do with them, or declare that they have forgotten how they should be used. Attempts to put on clothes proceed haphazardly. The order of dressing may be completely wrong: pullovers are put on before a shirt or blouse, pants after trousers, shoes before socks. Garments may be tried on upside-down, the wrong way round or inside out: they may not even necessarily be related to the correct body part. The person may endeavour to put their legs into a blouse, or their pants or cardigan over their head; they may try to put on shoes ankle first. Even if the person is helped to get one arm in a shirt, they may still struggle ponderingly to insert the other arm; and even if clothes are laid out in order, they may still not achieve the correct dressing sequence. In general, dressing is a lengthy, hit-and-miss affair for people suffering from this type of dyspraxia. They may stumble upon the correct procedure, and surprise themselves in the process, but then be unable to repeat the success.

The success rate may be higher in less severe cases, but the person still hesitates about which garments to put on next, and how exactly to get it on. Easier clothes such as socks or pullovers (though these, too, may be difficult) might be donned ably, but more complicated items may prove more problematical. Shoe laces, ties and some types of buckle remain obstacles even in mild cases.

The difficulty is not one of clumsiness or maladroitness. Buttons, zips and bows may cause problems, though the source of the perplexity is not the fine motor co-ordination required, but rather knowing which bits to relate to which and in what way. This applies to the dressing, overall. The basic disability appears to be a loss of control over the proper spatial–motor requirements required for the task, giving difficulty in orienting parts of clothes to parts of the body.

This disability is connected with both right and left hemisphere lesions. De Ajuriaguerra *et al.* (1960) found it in nearly 22 per cent of the right, nearly 4 per cent of the left, and 20 per cent of the bilateral lesion patients reviewed by them. It may co-occur with dysphasia, visual–perceptual problems and the common sequelae of these broader categories. These include problems of spatial orientation, constructional dyspraxia, spatial dysgraphia, dyslexia and dyscalculia, clock-reading, body part naming, and so on. The disability may be complicated further by hemiplegia, hemisensory loss, hemineglect, visual field defects, ocular motor disorders and in frontal lobe involvement with attentional and planning deficits. Postural and balance defects may also contribute to the picture in some cases, especially for lower extremity dressing. Adequate assessment must sort out the difficulties due to the central perceptual-motor disability, from the effects of these possibly co-occurring secondary factors.

What is Dressing Dyspraxia?

While it is generally agreed that people do exist with the problems described above, there is disagreement about whether the term 'dressing dyspraxia' is apt. The appropriateness of the label *dressing* and maintaining that it is a *dyspraxia* have been questioned.

The label *dressing* is arguably inappropriate from several angles. The different dyspraxias are subdivided according to the assumed disrupted *underlying process*, and not according to individual derailed actions. Gait dyspraxia was objected to because it was unlikely that a dyspraxia could exist that involved only one function of the legs. Likewise, to suggest that there is some discrete process — dressing — that is acquired and executed independently of all other processes is misleading. One does not speak of a 'making-a-cup-of-tea' or 'lighting-a-cigarette' dyspraxia independently from ideational dyspraxia, nor a 'wrapping-a-parcel-up' dyspraxia separately from callosal dyspraxia.

Following this argument, one would view dressing dyspraxia as only one manifestation of a more general disorganisation, which might include feeding and grooming difficulties, as well as failure on specific tests such as solving mazes, block design, object assembly and drawing. Those studies that claim cases of a discrete dressing dyspraxia can generally be criticised for their limited assessment approach.

The use of the word dyspraxia has also been considered as misapplied in this context. The label dyspraxia is deemed to imply a higher cortical motor disorder, with a dissociation between automatic and volitional performance, and a difference between performance to command and imitation, with and without real objects. The strict accuracy of this view has been questioned in several places in this book, but essentially the distinction holds. Further, each of the separate dyspraxias are characterised by specific error types and combinations not shared with other dyspraxias or other disorders.

None of these features holds exclusively for all cases of dressing dyspraxia. Neither do the problems evidenced by the person with so-called dressing dyspraxia fit neatly into the error patterns shown in other dyspraxias. The closest correspondence would be to constructional dyspraxia, a point taken up below.

It is contended here that dressing dyspraxia is not a specific, unitary disorder, but that it is one manifestation, among many, of other underlying dysfunctions. These relate chiefly to constructional dyspraxia and body scheme disorders. Several studies (Williams, 1967; Baum and Hall, 1981; Warren, 1981) have demonstrated a correlation between results on constructional tasks and the presence and prognosis of dressing difficulties. None of these studies used detailed constructional tests (copying simple drawings or geometric shapes; block and stick design), nor did they use sophisticated error analysis and scoring procedures. In fact, one criticism of them would be their simplistic error analyses. More careful comparison of errors on constructional tasks and dressing might well disclose greater commonalities.

The same studies, and others (De Ajuriaguerra *et al.*, 1960; Brown, 1972, for review; and Hartje *et al.*, 1975), have closely linked dressing problems with visual–spatial disorders and so-called body schema disruption. Thus, some patients have problems not only of relating clothes to themselves, but relating to the visual–spatial environment overall. They might lose themselves in the ward or at home, perhaps being unable to describe familiar routes, even with the help of a map, or they may not be able to complete simple mazes.

The idea of associating dressing difficulties with body image disorders deserves more detailed comment. Body image or schema is as abused a term as dressing dyspraxia (De Ajuriaguerra and Stucki, 1969; Poeck and Orgass, 1971; Frederiks, 1985). Many texts erroneously present it as a unitary datum, whereas in actual fact it is the product of many interacting variables. The developmental implications of this are mentioned in Chapter 7.

The label of impaired body image is usually applied after the person fails in one or a variety of tests purporting to measure body schema. These include right–left discrimination, finger recognition, and pointing to or naming body parts. However, a dual criticism of these assessments is possible.

First, the claim that such measures test body awareness appears to be an artefact of employing them only in relation to body parts. In personal experience, people who have difficulty indicating left–right on themselves have a similar problem indicating it on others, and more importantly on non-(human) body images such as houses or birds. Further, they have difficulty with other spatial pairs, such as top-bottom, front-back, east-west (for example, on a house, pointing out the top window or the back door, and so on). Those who fail at body part naming or pointing produce similar mistakes on indicating parts of a pictorial or model house, car or cow. People diagnosed as having finger agnosia, and thereby supposedly body image disturbance, likewise fall down on analogous non-body tasks — for example, finding the different coloured points of five-pointed stars, or pointing out the features of a complex geometrical figure.

Second, if it is accepted that similar errors occur on these tests in situations other than on body image assessments, it is clear that they must be measuring something beyond the hypothetical construct of body schema. The two main and general factors appear to be either language functioning or/and visual–spatial performance. General intellectual or attentional deterioration presents a third possibility. Hence, failures on right–left discrimination, body part recognition and the like, must be viewed in the context of the person's scores on language testing, visual–spatial tasks and general cognitive function.

These observations from personal experience are shared with Poeck (1975) and Poeck and Orgass (1971), who report experimental data to support the contentions. Warren (1981), in an evaluation of her data, pointed to certain skewing factors in the test of body perception used by her. One item involved drawing a human figure. Clearly, this may be influenced by motor as much as perceptual dysfunction.

Additionally, body image and dressing skill testing can be influenced by other consequences of brain damage. Inattention, neglect or denial of one side is an obvious feature to look for. So also are visual field deficits. The effect of these deficits is not simply to cut off one part of external or internal space. If one half of someone's world is missing, then the other half has to be reorganised to accommodate reality (see p. 81). This is one possible explanation of the complex disorder that often results from a seemingly straightforward and isolated defect.

Certain error types in ideomotor dyspraxia (p. 36) have also been mentioned as possibly misleading testers to an assumption of disturbed 'body-image'. In some cases, sensory or motor extinction and bimanual co-ordination may be underlying factors in impaired performance.

Clinical Implications

From what has been said above, it is clear that identification of a dressing dyspraxia should not be an end-stage in diagnosis but merely the start of assessment and rehabilitation efforts. Dressing disability needs to be further investigated to ascertain the underlying factors producing the person's problems. To say that disturbed body-image is the underlying cause is equally vague and misleading.

Behaviour must be examined within the framework of known visual–spatial and visual–motor deficits. Test results must be interpreted with attention to what skills are actually being tapped. Ideally, differential diagnosis should be made only after comparing verbal with non-verbally conducted tasks, visual–spatial with motor tasks, and dressing with non-dressing performance. The latter might include 'away-from-self' exercises, such as object assembly or perceptual matching, and also towards-self behaviours like feeding, grooming or body-part matching. More pertinent assessment should enable more specifically directed therapeutic intervention. Some points concerning rehabilitation are taken up in Chapter 8 on therapy.

The last word has not yet been said on visual–motor dressing difficulties. Though it represents an identifiable area of functional breakdown, the label 'dyspraxia' is misleading because it is not a higher motor planning disorder in the generally accepted sense of the word. Even those who originally coined the label did not envisage it as being restricted to praxic dysfunction. The label 'dressing' is also inappropriate since cases of isolated dressing disorder are rarely, if ever, found. Definitive answers will be found when the development and operation of actions in personal space, and the interaction of visual–spatial and motor functions in controlling these, are fully understood.

7 DEVELOPMENTAL DYSPRAXIA

Of all the areas for discussion in dyspraxia, the developmental type remains the most ill-defined. While agreement exists on what it is in general terms — usually centring around some notion of clumsiness or lack of motor skill — consensus is hard to find when it comes to specifics.

Is developmental dyspraxia (DD) a unitary phenomenon, or does it show itself in different ways from one child to another? Are there qualitatively different developmental dyspraxias? How does it stand in relation to other (developmental) motor disorders? Is it only a motor disorder, or must an understanding of DD also embrace perceptual development? Is DD even a delineable disorder? What is its relationship to such notions as minimal brain dysfunction and learning disabilities?

It is almost impossible to impose order on the diversity of answers offered to these queries in the space of one short chapter and still do justice to the many valid views. The aim here is to give a brief introduction to a vast and controversial field.

The chapter will summarise the salient features of DD, about which there is relatively general agreement. Through an examination from a more theoretical point of view, it is hoped that a clearer understanding will be gained of what should be looked for in identifying and treating DD. Based upon this, the manifestations of DD will be examined in two broad areas, limb and constructional dyspraxia. Finally, management issues are considered.

Defining Developmental Dyspraxia

The following remarks on DD find relative consensus from clinicians and from the literature (Walton, Ellis and Court, 1962; Ayres, 1973, 1979; Arnheim and Sinclair, 1975; Gubbay, 1975; Gordon and McKinlay, 1980; Cermak, 1985):

1. Central to DD is a disorder in motor function the affects that acquisition of new motor skills and the execution of those already learned. Typically, acquisition is a slow, effortful business and generalisation from one skill to another is poor or non-existent;

2. The motor disorder results from dysfunction at higher levels of

CNS operation. It is not explainable on the basis of poor physical strength, nor impaired primary sensation; it is not a result of straightforward maturational delay that will be automatically corrected with time; it is not due to any bodily deformity; and children with DD do not stand out as abnormal on conventional neurological assessment, but frequently they evidence soft neurological signs;

3. DD is not a unitary disorder: different children show varying profiles of disability. De Ajuriaguerra and Stambak (1969) speak of constructional, facial, ocular, postural and object dyspraxias. Aram and Nation (1982) discuss verbal dyspraxia, though Guyette and Diedrich (1981) call for a more rigorous examination of what exactly constitutes developmental verbal dyspraxia. Cermak (1985) discusses evidence supporting a distinction between a planning, conceptual dyspraxia and an executive one;

4. There appears to be a sub-group of children (they may even be the majority) who fail not only on motor tasks, but also on perceptual ones (tactile and visual). Hence, it is usually more accurate to speak of a perceptual–motor, or apractagnosic, disorder. Some workers (for example, Ayres, 1973, 1979) even view the prime underlying defect in DD as a lack of sensory perceptual integration;

5. Diagnosis depends not only on the severity of the central (perceptual–) motor dysfunction, but also on the demands placed on children by their environment, the social acceptability and tolerance of their 'errors', and the child's ability to cope emotionally with the problem. Hence the disability may not surface until particular demands overtax the impaired motor planning and execution system. For example, learning to write at school, piano or ballet lessons, or when joining friends in football or sewing;

6. Because of the centrality of perceptual–motor functioning to development in general, its disruption affects widely different areas — at home, learning to dress, to feed, open/close jars, enjoy play activities or tidy up; at school, learning to write, draw, participate in physical education; in the peer group, being able to join in with play activities without ridicule; the perceptual dysfunction, if present, may further affect reading, numeracy, and a host of other activities;

7. Inability to cope with demands may lead to emotional difficulties from frustration, failure and low self-esteem. Cermak (1985) reviews the possibilities that the emotional and dyspraxic difficulties may share common underlying causes — for example, insecurity about personal and physical image, from poor perception of intra- and extrapersonal space, and poor differentiation of self as object and subject in the world.

8. DD may occur as an isolated phenomenon or be associated with other disorders, either as a subpart of a broader syndrome, or as part of an overall dysfunction. Hence, it might occur as one aspect of so-called minimal brain dysfunction. In such cases, additional features might include hyperactivity or specific learning disabilities; it is seen in mentally retarded children, though DD occurs with the full range of intellectual ability and types of profile (low verbal but high performance, and vice versa); it can be found with other, frank motor disorders, for example the cerebral palsies (Abercrombie, 1964; O'Malley and Griffith, 1977);

9. A family history of DD is common, but not invariably present. The same goes for a history of perinatal complications (Gubbay, 1975);

10. It is wrong and misleading to think that DD is simply the same as an acquired adult dyspraxia in young children. The next section elaborates on the reasons why it is false to equate acquired and developmental dyspraxias.

In a more theoretically oriented look at the development of praxis, it is also hoped to highlight why there should have been so much confusion in the past about exactly what DD is, its relationships with other dysfunctions, and why there are considerable grey areas around the edges of the distinguishing points enumerated above.

The Development of Praxis

Children are not born with fully developed praxic ability. Praxis is an acquired higher cortical function. As such, it is not the simple product of motor maturation, though it is only through anatomical and physiological maturation that the climate for the emergence of praxis is created. But praxis does not appear automatically even when CNS maturity has achieved an optimum level, any more than language emerges automatically just because the prerequisite CNS sophistication to enable its development has been reached. Interaction with the external world is necessary for this to happen.

Thus, praxis can be seen as the product of a dual interaction — (1) within the CNS, and (2) between the developing CNS and the external world. This view has several implications for the understanding of praxis and, in turn, of dyspraxia, its assessment and treatment.

The nature of the internal and external interactions is not static. Praxis does not result from simply adding one stage of development to another, like blocks in a tower. Praxis at two years of age is not a miniature version of praxis at five years. Each new facet of praxic development expands actions quantitatively and, more importantly, permits qualitatively different units of action and forms of organisation. This is one reason why it is wrong to consider DD in the same light as acquired dyspraxia. It is not until 10 or 12 years of age in normal children that one can speak of praxis in the same context as adult praxis.

The Nature of Motor Development

Movement in the newborn child is dominated by primitive reflexes. The infant is an object of the environment and its own basic needs (feeding and sleeping). Motor maturation permits the gradual freeing of the body from these involuntary, reflex-induced reactions and paves the way for potential self-regulation of movement.

At first, this movement is global and poorly differentiated, without specific segmentalisation. Independent organisation of individual movement elements, and with this the seeds of praxis, is not possible until constituent elements of movement can be differentiated out of this global activity. Trevarthen (1984) details the advances made in studying just how early germs of later actions can be discerned. Establishment and differentiation of motor control proceeds in a well-ordered fashion — from head and neck control, through the trunk and out to the limbs. Limb control also proceeds in a well-ordered fashion from proximal to distal. The behavioural correlates of this are the progression from lying to upright position, and from gross to fine movement control. Motor maturation also brings greater control over speed, force, precision and co-ordination of movements.

However, fine motor control is not yet true praxis. Praxis has not been acquired simply because a movement has been observed. It (or true action, as opposed to basic movements) is established only when the child is capable of organising these basic movements and realising new possibilities of action, by combining and recombining them. Praxis begins when movement is freed from basic affective–physiological determiners and is cognitively controlled, that is, when higher cortical command is possible over more primitive levels of movement origin, when emotional, visceral and reflexive actions have given way to the habitual, and when the volitional, unco-ordinated, non-purposive movements are replaced by symbolic, purposive and operational actions. Piaget (1936, translation 1977, p. 447) emphasises the higher, intellectual superordinate nature of praxis and gnosis when he concludes that '. . . intelligence constitutes an organising activity whose functioning *extends* that of the biological organisation, while *surpassing* it owing to the elaboration of *new structures'* (emphases added).

Action is not only a motor operation, though. Action occurs in space. To begin with, there is a non-differentiation of spatial perception in the neonate, parallel to the non-differentiation and global nature of motor activity. The body is not perceived as being separate from external space. Later, but still primitive, movement continues to take place in intra-personal body space, with the self as reference. External space is only seen as a continuation of self and not as having an independent existence outside of immediate bodily experience. A true division of intra- and extrapersonal space evolves only with the achievement of the concept of object permanence and the realisation that the self is only an object among objects in the world that is capable of acting on other objects, or being acted upon by them.

This differentiation has parallels in motor development, in that it is only with the emergence of distal control and the capability of manipulating the external environment, that the stage is set for the development of object awareness and external space as independent from one's own body. It is in the interdependence of action and perception, praxis and gnosis, that their common origins and subsequent close links in normal and abnormal functioning can be seen.

In early development, action and perception have an almost symbiotic relationship. Initially, extra- and intrapersonal space, and action and perception are one. Only gradually do these reference points become separately organised. So-called body image does not develop through spatial and haptic perception as a single datum, separate in itself. Neither does the perception of extrapersonal space develop in this way. The multiple sensory experiences necessary for the development of the awareness of space and self in space are dependent on action. 'Space is meaningless apart from an acting body' (De Ajuriaguerra and Stambak, 1969, p. 445). Conversely, however, action is meaningless and ineffectual without spatial reference. Body image and spatial perception develop out of sensory experience, but sensory experience comes from inter*action*. Thus, the body is both the object and subject of experience. It is out of this continual dialectic that praxis and gnosis evolve. This ongoing organisation and reorganisation in the light of new data has been expressed in another way by Piaget (for example, 1977) in his paradigm of accommodation and assimilation to maintain equilibrium.

Anatomical–Physiological Correlates

This view of the development of praxis and gnosis from a largely undif-ferentiated, visceral–reflexive mode of organisation through more differentiated stages to voluntary control, has anatomical and CNS organisational correlates.

Yakovlev and Lecours (1967) established three zones of brain that myelinate at different stages and rates, corresponding to areas of CNS that are involved in primitive reflex activity, through to differentiated higher cortical function.

It has long been known (Flechsig, 1901) that myelination of the cerebral cortex also proceeds in a sequential hierarchical manner. Early myelination occurs in the primary motor and sensory (somaesthetic, auditory, visual) zones. These have extensive subcortical interconnections. In contrast, the latest zones to myelinate are in tertiary association cortex, zones that have predominantly cortical–cortical connections.

These facts are also reflected in the locus and distribution of CNS control of movement and action. Initially, organisation is at a spinal cord and brainstem level. Gradually, this progresses to involve midbrain and primary cortical zones. When cortical control begins to predominate it is at first diffuse, without lateralisation or specific localisation within one hemisphere. Parallel to the differentiation and specialisation of action behaviour, there is a move to specialisation of function both between the cerebral hemispheres and within each separately.

For these reasons, cerebral trauma in childhood does not give the same symptoms as would damage to equivalent areas in adults. It is also one reason why radiographic or electro-encephalographic searches for localised abnormalities (for example, Knuckey, Apsimon and Gubbay, 1983) associated with dyspraxia, or any other developmental dysfunctions, are likely to produce equivocal findings.

The Triune Brain

The view that there are three fundamental levels of development, organisation and operation in the CNS finds support from many sources. Although using different approaches and labels, several workers have arrived at a view of a triune brain.

Pavlov (see Luria, 1973) spoke of unconditioned reflexes, conditioned reflexes and the second signal system. Yakovlev and Lecours (1967) spoke of median, limbic or paramedian and supralimbic zones. McLean (1972) (on whose schema Brown (1977, 1983) bases his discussion) spoke of a protoreptilian, a paleomammalian and a neomammalian brain.

Brown speaks of a sensori-motor level, where visceral and reflexive activity at spinal cord and brainstem level predominates. A limbic–cortical level follows, linked with control intermediate between the previous non-purposive, extrapyramidal stage, and the succeeding purposeful, neocortical stage.

The emergence of neocortical control corresponds with the development of more individuated, segmentalised action, progressively more focused on the distal extremities. Hand preference appears at this stage and action begins to be perceived as taking place beyond the body. It is this potential distance (psychic and topological) between action and objects and self that hails the possibility of purposive behaviour.

Brown (1977) introduces a subdivision into the neocortical level, called the asymmetric–symbolic stage. 'Asymmetric' denotes the establishment of true lateralisation of function, 'symbolic' signifies the presence of truly representational, symbolic thought. It is at this stage that action, that is, praxis, finally achieves an independent status in the world, tied neither to reflexes, body space, nor the here-and-now.

Praxis also has a vital interactive role with language at this stage. Initially, action helps to create the new space and awareness within which language can develop. But, importantly, language in turn becomes capable of directing and re-presenting action. Through language, action planning can be made independent of time and space (see Luria and Yudovich, 1956/1971; Vygotsky, 1934/1962; p. 136).

These three levels of organisation as envisaged by the different workers, must not be thought of as operating separately and becoming defunct once developmentally superseded by another level. On the contrary, as Brown (1977, p. 73) summarises: 'Action is not simply a concatenation of movements linked up temporally, guided by concepts or an "action-plan" and adjusted along the way by hypothetical sensory-feedback mechanisms; rather, it is a cognitive product realised over several levels with each level represented in every performance.'

Luria (1973, p. 99), expressing the same view, states: 'Each form of conscious activity is always a complex functional system and takes place through the combined working of all three brain units, each of which makes its own contribution.'

A description of the development of these levels does not simply document ontological development. In as far as each level is involved in the genesis of each action, the description of the levels and their interaction is also a description of the microgenesis of each action (Brown, 1977, 1983).

Management Implications

This view of the development of CNS functioning and organisation leads to several observations in the understanding of DD, especially regarding contrasts between it and adult acquired dyspraxia:

DD is Not a Miniature Version of Adult Dyspraxias. It is a disorder of an evolving CNS, not a mature one. It passes through qualitatively different stages, and so manifests itself differently at different times. The child with DD does not have a 'memory' and lifetime's experience of learned action to refer back to like the adult dyspraxic. DD is a disorder of the acquisition of learned, volitional actions; adult dyspraxia is the breakdown of established motor patterns and voluntary control (although one element in some acquired dyspraxias is the inability to learn or relearn new actions — see p. 36).

The implications of this for assessment and therapy include:

1. Strategies and procedures worked out for adults will not necessarily be directly applicable to children;

2. Assessment and therapy will focus on different aspects at different stages in DD;

3. This focus will follow a developmental pattern, and will not be related to recovery patterns in acquired dyspraxia. There are some, though, who feel that recovery in acquired cases reiterates the developmental sequence;

4. This last point has itself several implications, as follows.

Distinctions Deemed Characteristic of Acquired Dyspraxia May Not Hold in DD. Children with DD have difficulty in acquiring volitional control of actions and laying down motor automatisms. Thus, the hallmark of DD may be the absence of volitional control and smooth-running programmes in habitual actions. So-called islands of fluency (p. 92), the correct carrying out of actions on occasions and the facilitation of performance in certain contexts, may be completely lacking from the picture, though this awaits final confirmation in detailed single case studies, which are lacking from the literature on DD.

Early (pre)praxic development disruption will bear close resemblance to, and even be indistinguishable from, other dyskinesias of subcortical origin because praxis grows out of more basic movement control. This is in contrast to acquired dyspraxia where, traditionally, there is a distinction between cortical and subcortical control.

Vygotsky (see Luria, 1973) and Ayres (1973), among others, have emphasised the disruptive influence that can be exercised on the development of higher cortical functions by dysfunction at lower levels. There are many skills that, initially, require conscious effort or even tuition (dressing, writing, use of various utensils), but which are later carried out with little or no conscious attention to each segment or part act. This is even more applicable to certain advanced skills, such as playing musical instruments, dance routines or driving a car. Disruption to lower levels of organisation, an inability to elaborate planning at higher levels and the consequent inability to form and retain action programmes will mean that these behaviours are not achieved in DD.

This applies also to skills not traditionally thought of as voluntary, learned skills, such as walking or eye movements. They are not volitional in the sense that they have to be consciously learned or taught — though the latter might apply in cases of severe handicap. However, their initiation, manner of execution and control can be (and sometimes must be) raised to 'higher' levels of control. For instance, walking must be controlled consciously by the infant to negotiate round, over or through objects; it has to be controlled consciously if the examiner asks the child to walk on tip-toes or heel-to-toe. Children modify their gait to imitate various people or animals, or just for fun.

Another relatively firm distinction in acquired dyspraxia is between perceptual and praxic causes of poor motor performance. In childhood, with the common origins of praxis and gnosis in action, the division between these two sides of the same coin is problematical.

Implications for Assessment and Therapy

1. Action takes place in a visual–spatial, tactile world;
2. However, sensory experience comes only through action;
3. Assessment and therapy must reflect this;
4. True praxis is not to be found in primary sensory-motor skills;
5. However, early assessment and therapy must be directed towards these areas (strength, speed, precision, joint position, tactile localisation and so on);
6. True praxis is to be found in the ability to integrate and organise lower functions to achieve new ends. Later assessment and therapy must concentrate on this;
7. Another dyspraxic difficulty, once integration is possible, is the learning and automatisation of this integration. Later management must also examine and treat this aspect of DD.

Assessing Developmental Dyspraxia

Assessing a disorder assumes one knows what one is trying to describe and quantify. The vast range of views on DD has spawned an equally vast range of tests, scales, programmes and techniques purporting to detect and measure it. The proliferation is compounded by each professional group dealing with dyspraxic children having its own mushrooming set of assessments.

Thus, while commonalities exist, occupational therapists, physiotherapists, psychologists, teachers, speech pathologists and physicians each have their own approach. Given the added fact that normal praxis is a function of many interacting subsystems, which all need assessment, it is no wonder the field of evaluation of DD is more like a jungle.

Order can be imposed if one accepts that assessment will be a process of exclusion of other disorders, and an inclusion, that is, identification, of dyspraxic signs and symptoms. The recognition of the latter will vary according to the developmental context within which DD appears. Three broad possibilities can be identified here: a general planning and organisational problem, in which such children are described as having an overall disorganised lifestyle in their attention, thought-chains and social development, as well as perceptuo-motor behaviour (Ayres, 1979; Small, 1982); lack of integration in perceptuo-motor behaviour only, with normal development in other areas (Ayres, 1973; Gubbay, 1975; Gordon and McKinley, 1980; Henderson and Hall, 1982); and a relatively pure motor dysfunction. These categories are based on clinical descriptive data. Whether they truly represent varying manifestations of DD awaits experimental confirmation. Cermak (1985) sets out arguments in this direction.

The recognition of dyspraxic signs and symptoms also varies according to the child's age, since DD manifests itself differently at different times in development, and according to the sphere of behaviour within which different clinicians or educationalists are searching.

Thus, the physiotherapist is more interested in posture, balance and locomotion; the occupational therapist in manual and overall self-help skills; the speech pathologist in oral-facial aspects; the teacher in literacy and numeracy. However, these viewpoints must not be seen as isolated and exclusive of each other. The efficient treatment team will share its findings to gain a unified view of the child, its strengths and weaknesses, and to organise a pertinent, effective habilitation programme.

The Assessment Process: Exclusion

Medical Evaluation. This will exclude other causes of childhood motor impairment, especially reversible or degenerative conditions. Gubbay (1975) provides a thorough coverage of this. Directions of search will be for: neoplastic disease; metabolic disorders; degenerative conditions; neuromuscular disorders; and other conditions, such as cerebral palsy, hydrocephalus, acquired CNS damage (CVA, viral, bacterial, malnutrition, accidental/non-accidental injury), orthopaedic problems, and visual/ocular motor dysfunction.

Psychological Evaluation. This will exclude general mental retardation, autism, and behavioural–emotional and other social interactional problems. The possibility must be borne in mind that some psychosocial difficulties may be secondary to an underlying DD.

Primary Sensory-motor Evaluation. This will exclude problems of tone, strength, speed and sensation (including auditory and visual) as main causes of the child's motor impairment. In early development, DD may be indistinguishable from deficits in this region (pages 158 to 178–9). The basic motor ability tests of Arnheim and Sinclair (1975), and the Bruininks-Oseretsky test of motor proficiency (Bruininks, 1978) provide normative data for these basic skills on which later praxic development depends.

The Assessment Process: Inclusion

Recognition of dyspraxic behaviour in adult studies has been through documentation of unique errors and according to multiple input and output variables, for example: naturalistic observation versus test situation; with versus without real objects; habitual versus non-habitual tasks; isolated versus sequential tasks; tasks in personal versus extrapersonal space; meaningful (symbolic) versus non-meaningful (non-symbolic); actions centred on different body areas — axial, proximal, distal (hands, fingers, oro-facial); verbal instruction versus gestural instruction or imitation; gestural versus constructional tasks.

Dyspraxia, or different varieties of it, manifest themselves in different ways according to the permutation of variables used. However, compared to adult studies, there has not been so much attention paid to the effects of including different dimensions in the assessment of DD. Most approaches use isolated, non-habitual, non-symbolic tasks to gestural/imitation instruction in test situations. Since experimental data comparing different stimulus and response variables in DD assessment is limited, discussion of the above dimensions is implicit rather than explicit in the following account. Significant advances in the understanding of praxis development and its description can be expected when the above variables are taken into consideration. Cermak (1985) has reviewed the current status of such attempts.

To date, two complementary approaches have been used to identify DD by inclusion: quantitative and qualitative methods.

Quantitative Measures. These identify dyspraxics as those who fall below a fixed score-line on tests purporting to tap praxic ability. Gubbay (1975, 1978) is a prime example, defining as dyspraxic those children who fall below a certain percentile on tests such as number of hand claps while throwing a ball and time taken to post a set of shapes. Kools and Tweedie (1975) used quantitative scores on an adaptation of De Renzi *et al.* (1966) to define their dyspraxic group. Meyer-Probst, Heider, Cammann *et al.* (1980) modified the finger postures and movement test of Lesný (1978), labelling children dyspraxic if they fell below a particular score on a straight pass-fail basis.

Other workers (see Gubbay, 1975; Gordon and McKinlay, 1980; Henderson and Hall, 1982, for comparison and review) have considered children dyspraxic if they show specific profiles on general intelligence tests, or on batteries of tests that contrast verbal, perceptual and motor functions. In particular, low performance and high verbal profiles have been claimed to typify the dyspraxic, especially if low performance comes from poor scores on form-boards, object assembly tasks, block design, maze completion, and similar.

These approaches can be criticised on the grounds that DD is not likely to be the sole cause of depressed time scores, failure to imitate postures and difficulty on block designs. So, while they might identify some dyspraxics, they do not identify all — and they do not exclude other sources of failure, such as abnormal muscle tone, reduced muscle power, poor vision or poor comprehension of tasks. Furthermore, comparing scores across subtests of intelligence scales to exclude other causes has been shown to be unreliable. Not all dyspraxics show a low performance, high verbal profile, and neither are all children with this profile dyspraxic (Aram and Nation, 1982; Henderson and Hall, 1982; Conrad, Cermak and Drake, 1983). Some show a high performance, low verbal gradient; in others, considerable praxic difficulties in one area pass unnoticed in overall scores. DD occurs with the full range of measured intelligence.

Quantitative scores, even where they do correctly classify dyspraxics, are not very helpful as regards intervention. They do not indicate why a child is dyspraxic and nor, more importantly, do they demonstrate in specific terms how the DD affects the child's behaviour.

Ayres (1980) claims that different profiles on her lengthy Southern California sensory integration tests diagnose different developmental disorders. They encompass a range of activities considered by Ayres to contribute to normal motor function. The tests of visual and tactile perception, motor accuracy, midline crossing, hand–eye co-ordination, and so on, are interpreted against Ayres' sensory integration theory of motor development.

Ayres diagnoses DD (1973) as a disorder in integration of somato-sensory stimuli, in particular, through inspection of the scores on the somato-sensory tests. Hence, for Ayres, depressed scores on tactile integration were especially indicative of DD. She did not find that assembling a mannikin or drawing a human figure detected DD adequately, suggesting that these tasks are related more to visual than somatic perception. On the other hand, Conrad *et al*. (1983) and others have found the section from the battery on imitation of postures to be the most useful in identifying DD.

While such diagnostic tests have advantages over quantitative results on more general batteries (in that they point to reasons for failure and suggest areas for therapy), in the final analysis they are only as valid us the theory from which they are derived. For these reasons, quantitative measures are always best complemented by qualitative analyses.

Qualitative Analyses: Gestural

While not yet as refined as for adult cases, there are data available that point to certain errors as being specific to particular developmental dyspraxias. Controversy within the field is rife, and a full exposition of arguments for all the alleged DD types is beyond the scope of this chapter Compare, for instance, arguments over developmental apraxia of speech in Guyette and Diedrich (1981) and Aram and Nation (1982). The following outlines of gestural and constructional praxis concentrate on the less controversial areas.

Bergès and Lézine (1963, transl. 1965) provide perhaps the most thorough test of imitation of meaningless gestures (one and two arms, hands, fingers), standardised on three- to six-year-olds. They present quantitative scores and comparisons to related measures (right–left orientation, body part naming and identification, draw-a-man, mannikin puzzle) and also include a qualitative analysis. They note such difficulties as poor synchronisation of simultaneous movements of limbs; correct posture, but false orientation in space; postures related to intra- instead of extra-personal space; groping for postures, and so on.

Their test includes imitation of finger postures. Those who support the relevance of these feel that studying finger gnosis and praxis provides 'evidence delineating certain factors which underlie the emergence of skilled differentiated action and the development of the body schema using the hand as a microcosm' (Lefford, Birch and Green, 1974, p. 340). It is assumed that abilities to name, locate and move fingers in certain ways develop in a clearly definable and age-specific manner.

Meyer-Probst *et al.* (1980) found failure correlated with other measures of perceptual and motor skills, as well as factors from the general case history. Others have not found a definable pattern of finger localisation (Poeck and Orgass, 1964, 1971; pages 152–3).

Kaplan (1977) summarises her work on gestural development, emphasising the qualitative changes in the performance of normal children at four, eight and twelve years. She asked children to gesture the use of various everyday objects. Identifiable response modes characterised attempts at different ages:

1. Up to four years: (a) pointing to the area where the action takes place; (b) manipulation of the object of the action, for example, pointing to the mouth when asked to gesture how the drink a glass of lemonade; holding the face when asked to show how to wash it;

2. Four years: body part as object (p. 30) begins to predominate;

3. Eight years: (a) development of the correct hand posture for holding the absent object; (b) but the hand is still held against the object of the action, allowing no space for the imagined object; (c) there is persistence of body part as object when demonstrating everyday objects in movements performed on the self and if the object of the action other than the own body is available (for example, pretending to hammer in a real nail);

4. Twelve years: (a) refinement of pretend holding postures to accommodate the size, shape and distance of the absent implement from the site of action; (b) greater tendency to act out the whole context in which the object is used.

Overton and Jackson (1973) also demonstrated a clear developmental sequence in gestural representation in the normal three- to eight-year-olds studied by them. In addition to the developmental sequence, reflecting that of Kaplan (1977), they found that, in actions directed towards the self, there was symbolic representation of imagined objects earlier than in actions directed away from the self.

Applications to Non-normal Groups

Cermak, Coster and Drake (1980) and Conrad *et al.* (1983) applied tests and error evaluations based on Kaplan (1977) to learning-disabled nine- to 13-year-old boys (high performance, low verbal IQ with reading difficulties versus low performance, high verbal profile).

In general, their findings reflected the findings of Kaplan (1977) and Overton and Jackson (1973) indicating the use of less differentially articulated, developmentally more primitive gestures in learning-disabled compared to normal boys. However, differences between groups were not uniform across subtests. This may be due partly to the composition of the experimental groups, which consisted of learning-disabled rather than specifically dyspraxic subjects. Other age groups, and groups or individuals, with different overall profiles may show quite different results. However, the relevance of Kaplan's dimensions was confirmed, in that variations occurred along them between the younger and older, and between the learning-disabled and normal children. The findings also revealed significant data for the hypothesis that gestural and verbal behaviour develop from a common sensory-motor substratum (Kaplan, 1977).

Conrad *et al.* (1983) found data suggesting optic–spatial and dynamic planning as two separately controlled aspects of motor production. They also suggested that spatial and symbolic components may not be separable before full CNS maturity.

These studies emphasise the multifactorial nature of DD and the variability of performance, even within a relatively narrowly defined area of learning disability. They also underline the paucity of knowledge in the area and the need for more intensive and principled research.

Assessment of Constructional Praxis

More than in any other area of praxis, constructional praxis, defined as the ability to manipulate objects in space under visual guidance, is rooted in visual–spatial perception and visual–motor control. It depends on the perception of objects, their form, size and colour, and the permanence of this form independent of the angle or distance of viewing. It also depends on the ability to perceive the relationships between different objects and parts of objects within the visual–spatial sphere, that is, distance, relative size and shape, reciprocal properties (pen to pen top; one part of a jig-saw to another; shapes to form-board), and so on.

Constructional praxis is predicated on the perception of spatial relationships not only for conceiving the end-goal of an action, but also for the visually controlled experimentation that goes into learning how to achieve that goal, and the visual guidance necessary in its execution. The picture of a child experimenting with different ways of how to post a shape through the appropriate hole provides a cameo of the acquisition of constructional praxis. The motor execution is dependent on visual guidance and perception, but at the same time developing perception is dependent on movement control and the ability to manipulate the environment. This is but another expression of the dialectic between self and external world, perception and execution, between the body as 'object and subject of experience' (De Ajuriaguerra and Stucki, 1969), which are so vital in cognitive development.

Assessment of constructional praxis, therefore, must attend to the visual–perceptual input, motor determinants, and their combination in visual–motor performance. Numerous assessments exist that cover these areas. General intelligence tests contain subtests relevant to constructional praxis, for example, form-boards, object assembly and block design. Another widely applied test is the Frostig test of visual perception (Frostig, 1966). It deals with visual–motor co-ordination, figure-ground perception, perceptual constancy, perception in space and perception of spatial relationships.

Each of these separate tests and subtests cannot be discussed individually here (see Burr, 1984; Taylor and Warren, 1984). The examiner must choose the relevant items or sections according to the aspect of constructional praxis to be assessed, the age of the child, the purpose of the assessment, and the validity of the assessment procedure/material for tapping aspects of constructional ability.

Evaluation of constructional praxis can be divided into two main areas, namely, two-dimensional (2-D) and three-dimensional (3-D) construction.

Assessment of Two-Dimensional Construction

Two-dimensional construction tasks include form-boards, block and stick design, as well as a range of paper and pencil procedures, such as drawing and copying geometric shapes, copied and spontaneous drawings, and writing.

Form-Boards. These include tasks involving the insertion of increasingly complex shapes into the board, pictorial scenes where individual items can be removed for reinsertion, and shape-posting tasks.

The Wechsler Intelligence Scales for Children and Merrill-Palmer tests, among many others, include form-boards. Gubbay (1975, 1978) provides normative data for the time taken on shape-posting.

No standardised versions of pictorial form-boards exist, but these are particularly useful in observational assessment for gauging how far the child is able to utilise information from the picture as a whole in guiding positioning.

Block Design. These tasks, such as the original Kohs block test (Kohs, 1919), or modifications of it incorporated into other batteries, are tests of 2-D construction, even though the blocks themselves may be 3-D. Norms and interpretative data are available in the individual test manuals.

Stick Designs. These fall into the category of 2-D assessment. Although

there are no standardised tests for children, adaptations of adult procedures (page 59) might be used. Developmental checklists (Sheridan,
1975; Holle, 1976) usually include reference to the complexities of design
that can be expected of children at different ages.

Paper and Pencil Procedures. These provide an especially valuable means
of assessment. They permit a whole range of tasks that tap not only the
more purely visual–spatial aspects of construction, but also the use of
an implement to achieve the constructional ends, and a means of recording performance not so easily available for other constructional tasks.
For this reason, the use of grapho-motor performance in constructional
assessment is discussed in more detail.

Grapho-Motor Performance

Constructional dyspraxia may result from poor motor development, poor
visual–perceptual development or the inability to combine these two components. Evaluation of grapho-motor skills permits the assessment of
these three areas.

Motor Component. The use of a pencil involves distal control of an implement performing a task in extrapersonal space. General aspects of
the gradual distal differentiation of motor control and its development
into external actions have been discussed elsewhere.

Specifically related to pencil use, one can observe: the development
of axial control as a firm and correctly positioned base for limb movement; the quality of proximal limb control; and the differentiation of
fine distal control in pencil-holding and manipulation.

1. Grasp is initially of the top of the pencil, which acts as an undifferentiated extension of the arm.

2. Grasp proceeds bit by bit down the pencil; it gradually becomes
an independent tool to be manipulated by the hand, rather than a mere
extension of it.

3. Parallel with this, there is a change from everted palmar grasp to
a thumb-middle-finger-index finger prehension, at around three to three-
and-a-half years old.

4. Control of movement also develops systematically from being gross
and proximally initiated, to being a fine, distal co-ordination.

5. Initially, the unused hand displays a mirror image posture. The
disappearance of this with the emergence of bimanual co-ordination frees
the other hand for other activities, in particular steadying the paper,
holding the finger by details to be reproduced on a copy, and so on.

6. The emergence of hand-preference and hand posture can be observed for clues to laterality.

Details of grasp development can be found in most developmental scales, for example, Sheridan (1975), Holle (1976).

Visual–Spatial Component. Motor development alone is insufficient for copying or the spontaneous production of drawings. The prerequisite visual–perceptual framework must be present. Like motor skills, this develops along ordered lines. For a full discussion of the contributing factors, specialist works in this field must be consulted (for example, Piaget and Inhelder, 1956; Bower, 1977; Goodnow, 1977). Only a few of the central features can be mentioned here.

1. Appreciation of lines and angles. Early 'pictures' tend to be circular scribbles. Lines and resemblance to adult drawings appear only gradually (though for some time prior to this, children will have verbally labelled their diagrams and protested to adults for hanging them upside-down).

The first lines to appear tend to be top to bottom, and precede horizontal ones. Diagonals appear last. The articulation of angles to achieve proper joints and closure develops later still. The development of line and angle direction is closely allied to the development of shape perception.

2. Size and relative size. Disproportion of elements of figures one to another is a feature of children's early drawings. This refers both to elements of a single figure (windows to wall; arms to trunk) as well as one figure to another (car to house; flower to tree). A much later product of accurate perception and representation of relative size is the ability to create perspective in pictures.

The same underlying misperception of relative size can be seen in the child's attempts to fit outsize bricks into a small trailer, sit on a model horse, or in misjudgements when passing through holes or tunnels in play.

3. Relationship of parts to whole. While parts may show internal consistency — for example, house wall and roof the correct shape; chimney and door proportionately accurate — the accessories are not necessarily related appropriately to each other. The chimney may be on the side wall and the front door half way up the wall.

These 'errors' are closely related to the development away from a feature-by-feature reference system, whereby drawings are produced with elements in sequence, without reference to an overall end plan; or a constant reference point outside of the whole. Only later does correct alignment emerge.

The orientation of the picture on the paper is allied to this also.

Initially, the tendency is for an angled orientation on the paper. Once the child comes to interpret the bottom of the paper as 'ground', the tendency switches to have everything positioned in relation to this.

4. Representational plan. Especially in free drawing, as opposed to copying, the child has to have some form of representational plan to work to. The development of such plans goes hand in hand with the emergence of praxis, since voluntary, goal-directed behaviour must be based on some representational notion of the aim of the action.

Those who use the interpretation of drawings in the assessment of constructional and other praxis, argue that through the analysis of the child's drawing strategies and end products, insights can be gained into the state and extent of visual–spatial representational development. The gradual differentiation of individual parts in a drawing; the ability to relate these one to another in a *unified* whole, and the possibility of producing an external (graphic, gestural, verbal) representation of the internal 'plan', are seen as being parallel to the differentiation and (re)organisation that takes place in limb praxic performance.

Hand–Eye Co-ordination

Hand– (and foot– and body–) eye co-ordination is not a unitary phenomenon, but the result of many interacting processes. It depends on: adequate vision, eye movements and visual perception; intact primary motor function and haptic development; and adequate body awareness, itself a product of multiple interacting variables (page 152–4). Therefore, assigning a diagnosis of poor hand–eye co-ordination is not an end–stage in assessment of constructional dyspraxia, but a station on the way to discovering why there should be poor co-ordination. The reason might lie in any, or several, of the areas above, or, crucially for constructional praxis, in the inability to integrate and organise the collective data.

The development of hand–eye co-ordination reflects the refinement of both visual and motor systems and the increasing ability of higher cortical control to organise the basic components. Early co-ordination is characterised by gross movements and poor integration of motor and visual data, producing misreaching, clumsy grasping and imprecise release (Bower, 1977; Trevarthen, 1984). Thus the child misses the object it wishes to pick up or move, or knocks things over instead of lifting them; Setting objects on top of, or inside, each other is inexact.

The child's first graphic efforts do not show any apparent hand–eye co-ordination. They are a predominantly kinaesthetic rather than visual experience. The same behaviour can be observed in attempts to fit formboard pieces or to post shapes. Later, visual control helps guide the more efficient motor system in the acquisition of habitual tasks and the execution of novel actions. Later still, when habitual action programmes have been internalised, they can be performed without constant visual guidance. The 'automatisation' of action programmes and the carrying out of novel tasks remain problem areas in the child with DD and poor hand–eye co-ordination.

All construction tasks involve hand–eye co-ordination initially, and can be used to observe its development. A formalised procedure useful for assessing hand–eye co-ordination in the grapho-motor area is the Bender Visual Gestalt test, or one of its revisions. There are several methods for scoring it (see Lezak, 1983; Lacks, 1984), covering the reproduction of individual items; the layout of figures involving multiple shapes; and variables such as symmetry, angles, joints, distortion and rotation. Koppitz (1964) has analysed young children's performance on the test.

Most developmental scales include approximate ages at which children start to be able to copy different shapes. Some go on to cover letter-copying ability.

Assessment of Writing Skills

Writing is a special kind of 2-D construction that may be impaired in the presence of otherwise normal praxis. It is an arbitrary visual symbol system for conveying thoughts, feelings and ideas. Thus, cognitive, language, reading and auditory factors clearly contribute as much to learning to write as visual and motor elements. These areas must be covered in a thorough assessment of writing problems. Readers might consult reviews by Bradley (1983), Cicci (1983) and Margolin (1984) for a fuller discussion of these inputs. Discussion here is restricted to the constructional praxic aspects.

Dyspraxic Dysgraphia. This can be said to exist when the child can recognise letters and words and indicate from among a choice of shapes and letters the one they are aiming for, but are unable to write it properly, spontaneously or to dictation. Such a child is not assisted by copying (Figure 7.1), since the defect lies in the motor component or the integration of the motor and visual components, and not in the recognition or recall of letters *per se*. Dyspraxic dysgraphia may occur as an isolated phenomenon, but it usually appears as part of a more general deficit in visual–motor integration. Therefore, most children can be expected to display errors on other visual–motor tasks.

Dyspraxic dysgraphia affects writing at the individual grapheme level.

Figure 7.1: Copying From Blackboard by a Child Aged 6 Years 8 Months.
(a) Today is Tuesday; (b) Here is a little kitten. She is; (c) Here is a dog

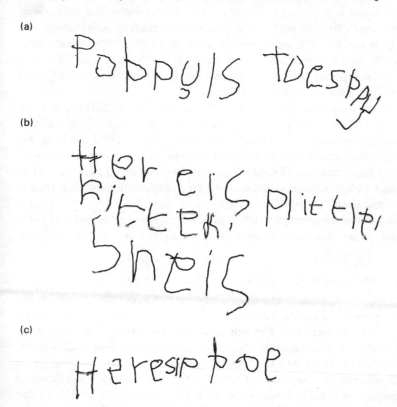

(a)

(b)

(c)

Directional and sequential errors can add further complication when the child starts writing words and sentences. Individual letters may be reversed or whole words and sentences may be written back-to-front; this is so-called mirror writing. Problems of direction interfere with individual letter writing, too. For instance, a tendency to move off in a clockwise direction can lead to reversals, or inversions on *c*, *e*, *f*, and the like. Starting a *b* with the *c* stroke might force the child into either a *p* or *d* when it comes to adding the down-stroke.

Sequential errors do not all stem from visual–spatial dysfunction. Auditory processing dysfunction can produce equally off-target words. Writing difficulties can arise from visual–spatial and auditory defects separately, but some children have problems from both. Therefore, assessment is not necessarily always one of deciding which factor is exclusively causing failure in writing, but in what proportions the different areas of deficit are involved.

Numbers and other tasks demanding accurate work can be impaired by dyspraxic dysgraphia — in geography, geometry and biology, for instance. Thus, it is legitimate to test children with poor numeracy skills for visual–motor disorder. Suspicion of such a disorder should be strong, especially when there is a marked discrepancy between a child's oral and written arithmetic performance.

In as far as there is frequently an accompanying visual–spatial component to the motor problem, one can speak of a spatial dyscalculia. If this co-exists with the dysgraphic element, then the child will have difficulty in organising figures into vertical and horizontal columns. Figures may be written out of sequence, multi-digit numbers in reverse order, decimal points inserted in the wrong place and fractions written upside-down. They may begin calculations from the wrong end; for example long-division from right to left, addition from left to right. Badian (1983) has reviewed the area of developmental dyscalculia.

Assessment of Three-Dimensional Construction

Like other forms of constructional activity, 3-D construction passes through recognised stages of development. Child development texts can be referred to for detailed coverage.

Towards the end of his first year, the child brings blocks together, tapping and rubbing them against one another. After that, blocks might be piled randomly into a box or other container, but proper construction does not begin until around 15 to 18 months. This starts when the child purposefully places bricks or other objects on top of each other. The number of bricks a child is capable of stacking increases with the degree of fine motor control and hand–eye co-ordination. Developmentally, vertical constructions precede horizontal ones, and 2-D comes before 3-D capability. Diagonal lines are more difficult than right angles. The step from 2-D to 3-D construction represents not only a quantitative leap, but is indicative of a qualitatively new organisation in the child's visual–motor development.

Assessment of 3-D constructional praxis has relied on formal tests and evaluation of the child's spontaneous productions with reference to developmental norms. Formal tests involve either assembly of objects, or copying 3-D block designs (see Figures 7.2 and 7.3 for examples) (Mitchell, 1976).

In the latter approach, scoring can be on a pass–fail basis or some kind of more sensitive score, for example, according to time taken;

Figure 7.2: 3-D Block Design to Assess 3-D Constructional Praxis

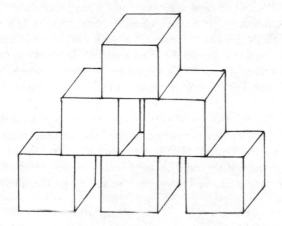

Figure 7.3: 3-D Block Design to Assess 3-D Constructional Praxis

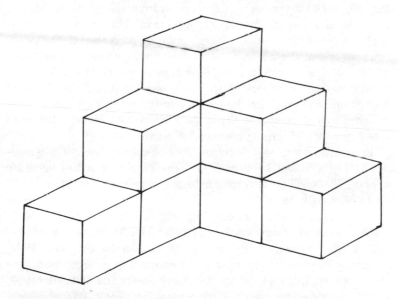

number of errors within certain specified areas; scoring model by model; gaining an overall reading. However, such scoring does not necessarily differentiate between dyspraxics and children with other movement disorders. A qualitative analysis of errors is recommended to make this distinction easier.

A variety of methods have been tried. Mitchell (1976) classified errors as omissions if the child neglected to include a block that should be present, or as substitutions if a block of a different shape or size was inserted. She called errors displacement if a block was placed on the wrong corner or section of the model. Others include as displacement the rotation of blocks through more than 45 degrees, separations and fragmentation of the model. Presence of rotation of the whole structure can be noted also.

Specific tests of 3-D constructional praxis include sections from general tests of intelligence mentioned on page 170, and Benton and Fogel (1962). Spreen and Gaddes (1967) obtained provisional norms for the Benton and Fogel test for children aged 6 to 15 years. Mitchell (1976) sought to provide additional norms in the age range five to six.

Summary

There is no shortage of tests purporting to measure development of praxis, even though they might not use the label 'praxis' as such. Indeed, in the field of DD the problem is sorting out from among the plethora of test material just which assessments provide valid descriptions of praxic ability, as opposed to more general motor or perceptual disability, of whatever origin. There is also a problem of finding reliable norms. Many of the tests if at all standardised, have been done so on limited populations, from the point of view of age range, socio-economic status, cultural background and numbers. Few of the tests currently employed were designed with praxis specifically in mind. Even those that were are based on often widely diverging concepts of praxis.

In order to bring some semblance of objectivity into the diagnosis of DD, further research will have to uncover more about the emergence of praxis. This will not only have to be in general terms, as clearly stated by De Ajuriaguerra and Stambak (1969), but also involve description of the qualitative aspects of development.

The comments of numerous earlier writers (De Ajuriaguerra and Stambak, 1969; Touwen and Prechtl, 1970; Henderson and Hall, 1982) regarding the poor delineation of developmental motor disabilities, one from another, still apply today. De Ajuriaguerra and Stambak (1969, p. 457) wondered 'whether it is not arbitrary to treat it (DD) separately before we have succeeded in distinguishing it within the more complex disorganisation of which it is part'. Touwen and Prechtl (1970, p. 88), in discussing the distinction between impaired and retarded co-ordination, note that 'This distinction may be very difficult or even impossible'. The same could be said for distinguishing between the many forms or

elements of minor motor dysfunction (which, nevertheless, may be causing maximum disability). The distinction is all the more difficult because
of the very nature of praxis. Separating minor primary motor disability
from DD in the early stages, especially only with tests of overall motor
ability (tapping, peg boards, and so on), may be questionable because
they both present as similar problems.

The work of Kaplan (1977), Cermak *et al.* (1980) and Conrad *et al.*
(1983) are steps towards distinguishing DD from other developmental
motor disorders along qualitative, cognitive and organisational lines. Such
work will also aid in the delineation of the varying manifestations of
DD. Quantitative scores will eventually have a place in assessment, but
are not likely to be reliable until the evaluation is made within a more
valid understanding of what DD entails. However, the fields of limb and
constructional dyspraxia and their differential diagnosis from other
developmental disorders are still in need of a thorough review akin to
that applied to developmental apraxia of speech by Guyette and Diedrich
(1981).

Its aims would be to examine just which of the countless features
claimed as characteristic of DD (poor rhythm, perception, reaching,
finger control . . .) actually are valid in formulating a differential
diagnosis, and which are merely hallmarks of general motor delay. It
would trace the genesis of various features of praxis and how they grow
out of earlier less specific types and levels of organisation of action. It
would establish how best to tap these fundamental features in assessment.

It is only when one examines motor ability in relationship to what
children are able to do with it in terms of cognitively imposed organisation, that a true picture of DD will be formed. The shortcomings in our
knowledge of DD and the consequent woolliness of defining criteria mean
that this is still no easy task.

Therapy

This section introduces the main areas and personnel involved in therapy
for DD. Further general points in dyspraxia therapy may be found in
Chapter 8.

A Multidisciplinary Approach

By its very nature as a multifaceted disorder, DD is likely to involve
therapeutic input from several directions:
   1. The physician will have dealt with medical differential diagnosis;

2. The physiotherapist will have assessed motor status;

3. The occupational therapist will have assessed self-help skills;

4. The psychologist will have evaluated overall cognitive development and relative strengths and weaknesses, in areas such as visual perception, attention, memory and numeracy;

5. The speech pathologist will have attended to speech and language factors;

6. If the child is of school age, the teacher (and perhaps also the remedial teacher) will have reported on school performance;

7. A social worker or counsellor may be involved if behavioural and emotional problems have arisen;

8. Most importantly, parents will have been partners in aiding the assessments, and will have highlighted the difficulties the disorder presents to them and the family, as well as to their child;

Because of the developmentally changing nature of dyspraxia, the input of these people will change, both as a function of the child's progress and of the demands placed on the child at different times. For the same reasons, prime responsibility for therapeutic content and direction will pass from one person to another.

Initially, the doctor will be the most important person, excluding underlying pathologies and referring the child to the relevant sources of help. Early on, the physiotherapist will play an important role in establishing basic motor control. The occupational and physiotherapist share the habilitation of gross and fine motor co-ordination. As skill passes to more complex everyday situations, the occupational therapist will be the leading person. If speech is involved, the speech pathologist may have a vital role. As speech improves and the main linguistic demands become reading and writing, then the teacher will take over.

Counselling is ongoing throughout therapy, and is especially important at the outset. However, if secondary psychosocial problems arise at any stage, the expertise of the counseller will be paramount. The psychologist's contribution will come to the fore if any behaviour modification programmes are deemed to be appropriate.

The prime importance of the child's family throughout cannot be overstressed. After all, it is they who spend the most time with the child, who are liable to be most concerned about the disability and who, after the child, are likely to be most affected by it.

The multifactorial presentation of DD also means that therapy will have to cover many areas, including: perceptual and motor training; speech and language; numeracy; literacy; environmental manipulation; attention; behaviour modification; medication for co-occurring disorders.

Each of these areas in turn will entail subdivisions. Perception might cover shape, size, relative position, direction, movement, colour or figure–ground discrimination. Motor training will deal with the posture and balance necessary for the firm base from which skilled movements are operated. It will cover gross and fine co-ordination, proximal and distal control, one- and two-handed actions, and movements performed in bodily and external space. It will coach relatively isolated actions, like copying a straight or angled line, picking up a cup, and progress to complex programmed activities such as dressing, writing, swimming or building model aeroplanes.

Clearly, with such a breadth of input and such a time-span of involvement, an overall co-ordination of activities is vital. From the family's point of view it is essential that:

1. There is one person with whom they can identify;
2. This person has an overview of the situation and future needs;
3. The person will be able to refer the family to the specialist concerned, if they alone cannot answer the family's queries;

From the therapeutic team's point of view, a central figure is advantageous:

1. To oversee progress;
2. To ensure that the right agencies are being involved at the right times;
3. To prevent any unnecessary duplication of input and, even more pertinently, to prevent contradictory input.

It does not much matter who in the team takes on this central role, as long as someone does. The co-ordinating role is as central to the problem as any perceptual or motor therapy, if relevance of direction and content is to be maintained.

The heterogeneity that exists among developmental dyspraxics will mean that no two children are likely to be exactly the same. Thus, while many children might require help in similar areas, the nature of that help will not necessarily be the same. Hence, it is wrong to think that there are off-the-hook programmes applicable to all children.

Certain implications can be drawn regarding therapeutic conduct and content. From the theoretical review:

1. Praxis is a higher mental, symbolic function;
2. Praxis grows out of, and is dependent on, many interacting strands, including: sufficient levels of arousal and attention; intact vestibular-labyrinthine systems; efficient pyramidal, extrapyramidal and peripheral nervous systems; intact sensory systems;
3. True praxis is seen as emerging only when the child is capable

of organising and reorganising the movement possibilities afforded by the maturation of these underlying systems into new actions. This goes beyond the level of basic reflex, tone, power and co-ordination, which are the domain of these contributing systems. As expressed by Brown (1977, p. 61): 'If movement can be taken to refer to behaviour in physical space — motility outside of cognition — then *action* occurs when movement undergoes a cognitive transformation';

4. Cognitive, volitional control of action removes movement planning from the constraints of the immediate environment. Action thereby achieves an independent status in the world, and the learning of new patterns of action and the conscious manipulation of that world becomes possible;

5. The emergence of true praxis from lower forms of control is a gradual process, in the course of which developing action undergoes continuous re-organisation and qualitative change.

This, in turn, led to certain implications for assessment and therapy. Two strands have been identified from the assessment review:

1. The development of basic motor skills;

2. The development of cognition and the order it is capable of imposing on underlying motricity.

Thus, dyspraxia is not to be seen as being hypo- or hypertonus, though either may be present in dyspraxia; neither is it manifested in a lack of basic postural reflexes, though this may be present too. Dyspraxia is not characterised by a depressed diadochokinetic rate on tapping exercises or poor performance on pegboard tests, though dyspraxics may score poorly on these. Lack of fine motor control, inco-ordination and dysmetria may also be found in dyspraxics but, again, these are not features of dyspraxia. While the dyspraxic child may be clumsy, clumsiness itself does not automatically mean dyspraxia.

Rather, dyspraxia is suspected when the child's execution of tasks is below that which would be expected on the basis of scores in primary motor tasks. Dyspraxia is probably the cause if the child is unable to learn an action which should be possible for his/her mental age, despite showing the presence of the component skills presumed to contribute to the carrying out of the action.

Dyspraxia must also be considered if the child is unable to organise component actions into an overall spatial–temporal plan. Impaired underlying motricity may interfere with the execution of actions, but dyspraxia is the disruption to the *organisation*, not the realisation of basic movements (though see Cermak, 1985, for suggestions that there is an organisational and an executive DD). Assessment and therapy must look to organisational integrity and quality and not just to performance skill.

That, though, is not the full story. Cognitive development is not an independent feature of development. It grows out of experience. If the quality of that experience is impaired, then cognition will be correspondingly involved. This is seen in the influence of lower level disruption on higher order processes (Ayres, 1973). Clinically, it is seen in the findings of perceptual and praxic difficulties in the cerebral palsied (page 157), a group traditionally thought of as suffering from only primary motor dysfunction. It is seen in any cases where there is experiential isolation.

The close relationship between the development of praxis and perception, which grow out of the same interactive experience, has also been stressed above. This bond finds expression in some alternative labels for DD, for example 'apractagnosia' or, emphasising the importance of bodily as well as external space perception, 'apracto-asomatognosic' syndrome (see De Ajuriaguerra and Stambak, 1969). The gradual differentiation of perception and execution have been assumed to reflect a gradual functional differentiation of organisation and representation in the CNS (page 159).

Therapeutic Considerations

This is not the place to consider fully those therapeutic principles that apply to remedial education and developmental intervention in general. Experienced clinicians will be well familiar with guidelines, such as following the developmental sequence, not expecting a child to acquire skills that have not been prepared for by ensuring the presence of the underlying prerequisite factors, or which are way beyond what any other child of similar mental age would be able to do. Other guidelines include establishing perception before expression, not expecting the child to express meaningfully contrasts in position, shape, meaning and so on until the child can perceive these same differences. This is not to say, of course, that the child does not learn to perceive partly through action.

Another general principle adhered to is to encourage strengths at the same time as one treats weaknesses, or tactfully drop one expectation in favour of another (for example, learn to run instead of to play tennis, or learn to buckle instead of lace-up shoes). These principles can be found in any general textbook on remediation. Works concerned more closely with the dyspraxic child include Johnson and Mykelbust (1967); Ayres (1973, 1979); Arnheim and Sinclair (1975); Gordon and McKinlay, 1980; Small (1982); Laszlo and Bairstow (1985).

Content of Therapy

Exactly what is included in any therapeutic programme will depend on the individual's needs. Some of the areas were already mentioned above. Central to tackling the dyspraxia will be the training of motor programming, accepting, of course, that perceptual, language, attentional and other motor disabilities might be part and parcel of the syndrome, and also require therapy.

Following the principle that praxis emerges out of basic motor functions, a motor training programme will cover these areas. In this, suppression of primitive reflexes and development of tone for maintenance of posture and balance will be a first priority. Proximal limb adjustments can be made with efficient axial control, and a reliable framework created for precision movements in bodily and external space. Gradually, with the development of distal control, gross motor action can undergo a progressive differentiation to increasingly finer movements. However, praxis is not achieved with the acquisition of basic motor control: it is predicated upon this. Basic motor control is exploited by higher cortical processes which permit organisation and reorganisation of the basic functions to achieve new levels of sophistication in action.

This takes place first in relatively immediate time and space, and perhaps involves only one limb. Through maturation, motor planning becomes increasingly more complex, both in terms of spatial and motor detail and projection into future time, and the role which language can play in planning. Eventually, the aim is that a child should be able to piece together a complex action such as screwing on a jar lid. The child should also be able to mentally conceive action plans comprising a series of complex movements directed towards a specific goal, for example, getting a biscuit out of a packet in the cupboard; writing a word; putting on a jacket.

With some severely disabled children, it has to be realised that this aim will not be reached. Even in non-dyspraxic children, it is often not until 10 or 12 years that such levels are attained.

Skills versus Process Training

The notion of praxis arising out of higher cortical (re)organisation of basic motor function raises important questions for therapy. A predominantly skills-orientated approach to therapy is adoptable in training or encouraging basic motor activities, because dysfunction at this level is relatively amenable to direct intervention. However, the picture is quite different when cognitive processes need to be encouraged or influenced. In this case, process-oriented therapy is required, dealing with operations (perceptual, motor and linguistic) that are assumed to underlie the acquisition and functioning of new levels or forms of cognitive organisation.

This represents a controversial issue in therapy. Can one train higher cortical functions directly? Naturally, those who have developed perceptual motor programmes under various labels to do this, claim that it can be done. Others hold a less strong position, maintaining that one can create the learning environment and provide the presumed necessary input, but that it depends on the individual child as to whether or not the vital cognitive leap is made. Yet others contend that only skills can be taught and that underlying cognitive processes are not open to therapeutic manipulation.

Therapists have worked with varying combinations of these hypotheses, regardless (see also page 197). Whole programmes have been devised based on such claims. However, as Small (1982, p. 155) rightly concludes, there is 'much advocacy, but little research', and intervention for dyspraxic and other learning disabled children still rests largely on faith and little on fact. Future research must improve not only knowledge about the development of praxis, but also of what is and is not effective in therapy, how strategies become effective and how progress can most efficiently be brought about and maintained.

For instance, many programmes include activities that are directed towards bettering the perception of body schema to improve praxis. Aside from the vagueness of what actually constitutes body schema (see p. 152–4), this therapy is usually coupled with some theoretical notions about why the approach might be useful, but next to no hard facts about whether it really is worthwhile. Some would argue that if an approach seems to work then it should be used, regardless of *how* it works. But even this is unscientific, since it has not been established exactly which factors in the therapy are producing the change. It might be improved perception of personal space, or sub-aspects of this, or factors totally unrelated to the specific content. Nevertheless, with these criticisms in mind, one can mention remediation approaches.

Therapeutic Programmes

Not surprisingly, there are as many different approaches to DD therapy as there are definitions of it. The number is swelled by variations on the commoner themes introduced by each therapist group and the introduction of their own idiosyncrasies. Certainly, such variation should be expected sometimes, since different therapists provide input to different areas at different stages; but one is often struck by the lack of integration, repetition and redundancy in many regimes. Lists and outlines of many of these programmes can be found in Arnheim and Sinclair (1975) and Burr (1984).

Some programmes are based on theoretical models of dyspraxia (not always DD). These are only as valid and reliable as the model upon which they are based. However, there are others that are not derived from any explicitly tried-and-tested theoretical basis, but which rest on a general philosophy of education, which is assumed to be applicable to normal and atypical development and by implication, therefore, would include DD. Yet other programmes do not claim to cover all the needs of the child, but concentrate on one area or stage of development presumed to be deficient in DD. Thus, one might find programmes for rhythm, body image or tactile-kinaesthetic perception, or literacy readiness (Johnson and Myklebust, 1967; Kephart, 1971; Ayres, 1973, 1979; Arnheim and Sinclair, 1975; Gordon and McKinlay, 1980). The danger is that sometimes they are used indiscriminately beyond the bounds within which the programme was originally envisaged.

Each of these points underline the need for the team to sit down and draw up a plan suitable to the individual's requirements, one that will receive ongoing review and that takes into consideration the child's progress and changing external circumstances. Such a plan must be founded on thorough and accurate diagnostic information. This may seem too obvious to mention, but it is not uncommon to come across children who have been tagged as being 'dyspraxic' on the evidence of limited assessment information and who have been entered into an off-the-hook programme without regard to their special needs. Clinicians should not be surprised that they are asking themselves why, in such cases, the child is failing to stride ahead, why therapy is taking an inordinate amount of time and why secondary psychosocial problems are arising.

Individual Programmes

Methods deriving from an overall philosophy of education that have been applied to clumsy children include the Rudolf Steiner and Montessori methods. While there are particular activities derived from these philosophies, their advantages lie in the overall attitude to the child and their problem, rather than in the specific content they offer.

Kephart (1971) evolved a system of perceptual–motor training as a way of encouraging academic potential and remediating learning disabilities. Through the use of balance boards, dancing and rhythm routines, trampolining and so on, Kephart aimed to foster balance and posture, locomotion, and contacting, receiving and propelling objects, upon which he felt learning was dependent. He emphasised visual tracking and figure-ground activities.

Johnson and Myklebust (1967) presented what they termed a psychoneurological approach to learning disability intervention. They drew on concepts and techniques from education, language pathology, psychology, psychiatry, neurology and biomedical engineering. Their principles and practices do not relate solely to so-called dyspraxic children, but also cover areas such as reading, arithmetic, social perception and language.

Ayres (1973, 1979) bases her therapeutic strategies on the premise that poor perceptual and motor function derives from lack of sensory integration. Hence, she includes techniques aimed at providing a variety of sensory experiences. For instance, to stimulate vestibular reflexes, Ayres has the child swing and spin in a net, travel in different positions on a scooter-board, or roll on a large therapy ball. In keeping with her proposition that function at a lower level of CNS organisation influences higher functions, most of the therapy is directed at stimulating spinal cord function and brain-stem and mid-brain processes.

Arnheim and Sinclair (1975) present their own programme of motor therapy for the clumsy child, drawing on several traditions. Their detailed procedures are not only designed for the professional therapist, but most can be integrated into youth club activities, general education and family life. Although there is some perceptual input, emphasis is on motor fitness, balance, locomotion, rhythm and temporal awareness, projectile skills and selected play skills.

Gordon and McKinlay (1980) bring together professionals involved with clumsy children, including occupational, physio- and speech therapists, teachers and psychiatrists. Each presents their possible contribution: Cahn and Hodges (1974) and Burr (1979, 1984) outline the approaches used by occupational therapists with dyspraxic children; Baker (1981) does the same for physiotherapy; Tansley (1980a, b) covers very much the same ground. The contents of these programmes owe much to the works of Arnheim and Sinclair (1975), Ayres (1973), Johnson and Myklebust (1967), Kephart (1971) and others.

Golden (1984) discusses certain controversial therapies such as megavitamin therapy, dietary manipulation, orthomolecular mineral therapy and others. Discussion of their application is centred around the so-called hyperactivity syndrome, but it is noted that these therapies have been applied indiscriminately to the whole range of learning disorders.

Clinicians will find abundant suggestions for therapy in the works referred to above, however unsubstantiated their efficacy might be.

However, one area of therapy, counselling, perhaps warrants a more detailed mention.

Counselling in Developmental Dyspraxia

There are three ways in which this is important.

Between Team Members. The counselling of one team member by another on their findings, approaches the problems encountered with the child. The ways in which members can mutually assist each other is most important. Strictly speaking, this is not counselling, but represents the vital liaison that must take place between involved parties.

Team Member to Parent. Counselling from team members to parents, and other relevant people associated with the child outside the immediate team is the second type of counselling. Each individual must communicate his role, findings, their significance, the intended intervention procedure and the role the parents are expected to assume in therapy. One team member should also have responsibility for explaining the overall situation to parents.

This person is required to explain the nature of DD and how it relates to the child's behaviour, including those aspects of which the family may be aware, as well as others which they may have overlooked. The team member must also inform the family on the possible consequences for school placements, progress, anticipated difficulties and how these might be minimised or avoided. They can reassure them that DD is not a deteriorating or life-threatening condition, and that it does not equate to mental subnormality, a fear frequently expressed explicitly or overtly. At the same time, they must speak realistically of the problems and what can or cannot be done about them. Most people are often ill-prepared for the long and dedicated work needed to help the dyspraxic child.

While maintaining a balance between anticipating expected difficulties and discouraging self-fulfilling prophecies, danger areas and times can be talked through. Starting school, moving to secondary education (Levine and Zallen, 1984) and choosing a job can be testing times in the academic career. Finding playmates, being accepted as one of the gang or realising parents' expectations may be sensitive areas in social life. Parents may need to be guided in modifying hopes that their child is going to realise their own ambitions as a great footballer, ballerina or musician, or even just coping with everyday life. Prudent alternatives can be put forward that build on the child's strengths. The same holds true when it comes to choosing a job, although years of adapting to and avoiding awkward demands at school may well have pre-decided the direction.

Developmental dyspraxia, like many other handicaps, can bring about disturbed relationships between family members. These are not confined to relationships with the dyspraxic child, but may affect life between the parents, the child and siblings, and other siblings and the parents. Parents' attitudes to their dyspraxic child may include over-indulgence, which leads in turn to stunting of the child's emotional growth or an inability to cope with the frustration of the disorder, and to sibling rivalry. This also opens up the danger of the child accepting the role of one who has to be assisted, that is, learned helplessness. However, the parents' attitude may be intolerance, exasperation, fright or anger, each of which can lead to the child's social and emotional isolation in the very place where they should be able to find acceptance — at home. Such feelings may derive from a sense of guilt, misunderstanding or through the perceived added burden of a 'difficult' child exposing tensions already inherent within the family. Dealing with these aspects is the job of the trained counsellor. Guilt and misunderstanding can largely be allayed if there is an initial and proper counselling from the therapeutic team on the causes of DD, as far as they are known, and its behavioural manifestations. The family needs to know that their child is not purposely scattering their dinner everywhere, that they are not lazy at learning to write or to dress themselves, and that they are not defying parental discipline by not putting toys neatly away. Thursfield (1980), Small (1982), and Hunt and Cohen (1984) have discussed the management of this area.

Team Member to Child. The counsellor might have a direct role in treating DD. As children mature and can verbalise their anxieties, this could involve direct psychotherapeutic discussion; otherwise it might be done through numerous indirect channels. Problem regions include the child's self-esteem and the possible alienation in home and school. In the latter, truanting full-time or from certain lessons (writing, physical exercise and art) may develop. One needs to be alert to the presence of psychosomatic manifestations of difficulties.

For further discussion of these aspects, ample information is available in the literature on all types of handicaps, as well as in the counselling literature. Regrettably, there are still too few guidance personnel qualified in this field.

Conclusion

One is more than aware that much has been omitted in this review of DD. An attempt has been made to narrow down discussion of dyspraxia to its more central features, on the one hand delineating it from the more global and undifferentiated definitions that abound and, on the other hand, broadening the conception out from those that see DD as being definable in terms of performance in one or two isolated behaviours.

The emergence and development of DD is seen in dynamic, gradually evolving terms. DD is seen as resulting from a failure at the higher cortical, conceptual-organisational level of motor control. The interdependence of praxic development with other major strands of CNS and cognitive development is also stressed in this view, particularly its dependence on, but growth beyond, basic motor development, its symbiotic relationship with sensory–perceptual function, and its eventual close links with language for action programming. The implications of this perspective for assessment and treatment have also been outlined.

The variety of views that have been used in defining DD mean that it has been largely pointless to discuss incidence, aetiology, prognosis, ratio of male-to-female cases and other aspects that should contribute to a proper appraisal. This does not mean that valuable points are not to be made about these areas (Gubbay, 1975; Gordon and McKinlay, 1980; Small, 1982; Knuckey *et al.*, 1983).

In summary, excerpts from a personal case are presented which cover some of the essential points made in the chapter. It especially illustrates: the early difficulty in differentiating between basic motor retardation and higher level dysfunction; how maximum difficulties arise despite minimum signs; the gradual emergence of a dyspraxic picture and the changing character of it as development proceeds and new demands are placed on the child; the long-term commitment of child, family and therapist in DD.

Case History

E.H. was referred to speech therapy at the age of four years and two months (4.2) by her health visitor because of unintelligible speech. There was nothing abnormal in the medical case history from pregnancy to time of referral. Her father had been late to start talking and an elder brother was described by the educational psychologist as hyperactive. Physical assessment, vision and hearing were normal. Quantitative assessments showed a developmental delay:

Stanford-Binet Intelligence Scale: At chronological age (CA) 4.2, mental age (MA) 3.4 (IQ 70–84)

Reynell Developmental Language Scales: At CA 4.2, comprehension age 2.6

However, further analysis of the profiles and information suggested that E.H.'s problems went beyond one of mere maturational lag.

Motor Development. Milestones for sitting, standing and walking unaided had been passed within normal limits. But her parents described her, and she presented as, a clumsy child — unintentionally destructive of things at home, a messy eater, unable to dress herself ably, and with poor balance. Although only living across the road from the clinic, E.H. was always late for her early morning appointment because of her slowness at eating breakfast and dressing.

On the coffee jar test (Gordon and McKinlay, 1980) at 4.2 years, she was unable to walk heel-to-toe; could walk on the edges of her feet only if hanging on to furniture; was unable to walk on tip-toe; could barely manage two hops; and showed no hand or foot preference.

While she could stack up to 12 2.5 cm cubes, she was incapable of placing bricks orderly on the table with each hand simultaneously. Trying to wind a lace round a reel, she ended up with it tangled round her hand. Bricks were threaded but, with much trial and error, stabbing took inordinately long. Arrows were copied but were unrecognisable as arrows without the models being available (Figure 7.4); the same applied to shapes and human figure copying (Figure 7.5). Despite this, she had no difficulty discriminating, matching and classifying shapes, nor on visual sequencing tasks.

Figure 7.4: An Attempt to Copy Arrows By E.H., Aged 4.2 Years

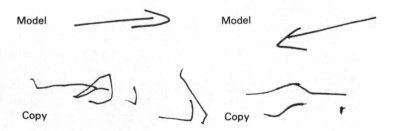

192   *Developmental Dyspraxia*

Figure 7.5: An Attempt to Copy a Human Figure by E.H. Aged 4.2 years

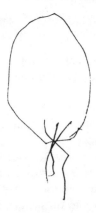

Speech and Language. E.H. scored below her age level in all areas of language development. At 4.2 years her unintelligible speech rendered expressive measures problematical. Utterances consisted predominantly of strings of three or four vowel–consonant syllables. The problem did not appear one of straightforward delay. With the exception of affricates (*ch*, *j*) and /f/, /th/ and /l/ sounds, she had a full sound inventory. Consonant–vowel syllables could be produced to imitation. Production of sounds in isolation was consistent and stable. However, both vowels and consonants sounds were unstable in connected speech and multiple repetitions of the same syllable, showing much distortion and sometimes apparent frank substitution. Repetitions and spontaneous speech were also highly dysrhythmic. Auditory discrimination of other people's speech was good. It was not until after about one year of therapy that she attempted self-corrections.

Her history is suggestive, so far, of DD in that:

1. There is an absence of hard neurological signs;

2. Intelligence is low average, but there are stark contrasts between different subtests. Perceptual tasks are up to chronological age, expressive scores severely depressed;

3. Muscle tone, power and sensation were normal but E.H. showed poor balance, posture and co-ordination;

4. Motor difficulties were even more marked when greater demands were made on temporal and visual–spatial planning.

E.H. is now eight years old. Since initial assessment and hesitation over whether her problem was one of straightforward overall delay or a more complex problem, a picture of clear DD has emerged. How and where it is most plainly manifest has changed over the years. When first seen, the problem showed itself in more basic motor skills (balance, gait), while more complex actions (bimanual co-ordination, copying, speech) were severely impaired or impossible. Through maturation and therapy, gross motor behaviour is now adequate and precision of movement is accurate, but she has great difficulty in organisation of movements in terms of (multiple) limb co-ordination and the sequence of elements within an overall action.

These difficulties are brought out on 2-D and 3-D constructional tasks. Tapping rhythms with one hand or foot, or alternately tapping hand-hand-foot-foot are barely accomplished. The dysrhythmic and sequential breakdown are heard in her speech on multisyllable words and in long utterances. Otherwise, her speech is approaching 100 per cent intelligibility.

DD has posed problems for her at school. Written work and constructional play (Figure 7.1 is by her) have been a constant source of failure, and she has had to stay down a year at school because of it. She has very good sight vocabulary in reading, reflecting her good perceptual attention, but has poor phonic skills which are portrayed in writing in poor grapheme–phoneme correspondence. The auditory sequential and constructional difficulties also make for poor spelling and written number work.

E.H. is described by her teacher as generally untidy and disorganised in all her motor activities. On the plus side, she has good oral language and is noted for her fertile imagination and narrative skills.

She is somewhat isolated socially because other children feel she disrupts their games by not playing properly. Living in an area with a strong cultural tradition, she was keen to learn dancing but, unfortunately, had to give up after failing to master even the most basic steps. The same happened when she switched to karate, though at least it suited her rough-and-tumble nature. Despite being an early riser, she continues to be late for appointments because of the length of time it takes for her to get ready. On arrival at the clinic, she takes several minutes to get off her satchel and coat, hang them on the chair, take out her homework and set it out on the table.

Each advance has been made only with the maximum amount of effort on her and her family's part. As new challenges are met, new problems arise. Life is never a smooth, easy running affair, and fatigue and ill health soon expose the precariousness of her gains. To date, the weight of therapy has been directed towards the assumed primary difficulties of motor co-ordination and action planning. Therapy will have to continue. The main input is now switching to a school- rather than clinic-based input, and a broader counselling and environmental approach to help her cope with the ever-present frustrations, social isolation and thwarted ambitions, as well as her schoolwork problems.

However, the question remains of whether therapy would have been so lengthy if knowledge of DD would allow (1) recognition at an earlier age, (2) analysis of subaspects of the syndrome, leading to (3) more pertinent and specifically directed intervention strategies and techniques which had (4) been subjected to well-controlled clinical trials to verify their (5) overall efficacy and (6) optimum area of disability to which they can be directed and (7) optimum age and stage at which they should be introduced.

To date, intervention has proceeded along lines dictated by general interpretations of developmental studies and clinicians' intuitions regarding the best time, type and place for therapy.

Over the past few years a small start has been made at placing remediation on a more objective footing. Future investigations must intensify the search for solutions to these points if involvement with DD is to be anything more than just a well-informed concern, and be placed on a relevant professional basis.

8 THERAPY

Therapy for dyspraxia does not take place in a vacuum but in the context of the person's injury and associated disabilities — be they physical, cognitive, emotional or social. It is influenced by the person's past experience. In addition, the availability of rehabilitative help, the individual's and the family's attitudes towards this, and the nature of that help will also have some bearing on outcome.

Most therapists have a set of working hypotheses which they use to weigh up the value of these factors in deciding on suitability for therapy, type of therapy (supportive versus intervention; short-term versus long-term, and so on) and prognosis. These hypotheses tend to be no more than heirlooms which have been handed down and, until recently, were little questioned. They make such claims as: the younger the person the better; the sooner therapy is begun the better; any therapy is better than no therapy; overlearnt skills will be more intact than those more recently acquired; and the bigger the lesion and the greater the number of disabilities, especially of perceptual ones, the poorer the outlook. Many more are listed in works on rehabilitation.

However, since serious investigations started into the validity of these assumptions, the picture has been shown to be considerably less straightforward, discussion of which is beyond the scope of this book. However, an understanding of the issues is vital if advances in therapeutic relevance and efficiency are to be gained. Studies on the significance of age, severity of insult, recovery patterns, the influence of therapy and so on, have been discussed extensively by Jennet and Teasdale (1981); Rosenthal, Griffith, Bond and Miller, J. (1983); and by Miller, E. (1984). Discussion of these points in relation to dyspraxia is conspicuous by its absence.

Another area beyond the scope of this chapter is a discussion of the practicalities in designing intervention programmes. Again, coverage of these is found in any textbook on rehabilitation — for example, Carr and Shepherd (1980); Diller and Gordon (1981); Golden (1981); Hopkins and Smith (1983); and Rosenthal et al. (1983). The application of these principles in choosing strategies, techniques and tasks in dyspraxia therapy is the subject of the remainder of this chapter.

General Considerations and Issues

Dyspraxia will seldom be an isolated problem with remediation directed solely to it. It is possible that there will be co-existing disorders of visual–spatial functioning (field defects, neglect, agnosia and so on); language; hemiplegia or paresis; memory and attention; and affect and motivation. Rehabilitation of dyspraxia will be dependent on and complementary to improvement in these other areas. The degree to which dyspraxia becomes a focus of therapeutic attention will also depend on several factors: the objectively assessed severity of the impairment might be one. However, functional impairment does not usually equal the degree of impairment that would be expected from the alleged objective score. This can derive from the cumulative effects of the many disabilities with which the person may be presenting. On the other hand, it may be totally unrelated to this. It is a well known phenomenon in all fields of disability that two people with apparently identical defects experience quite different levels of difficulty. This is not restricted to neuropsychological impairment, but applies equally to physical disability or deformity, pain perception and grief reactions.

Likewise, different people will have varying lists of priorities regarding which disorder they would most like to have 'cured'. For one person mild dysphasia may be of far greater concern than the severe constructional dyspraxia from which they suffer; another may not care at all about their hemiplegia and memory problems, but only that they cannot get out their cigarettes and light them.

The patient's future intentions and the family's and therapist's hopes for him will also dictate rehabilitation priorities. Is the ultimate aim a return to previous employment, alternative employment, sheltered accommodation or continuing care? These aims will make corresponding demands on therapy content and direction. When designing a programme, it must be asked, 'Therapy of what and for what?' Simply entering patients into non-specific and general programmes leads only to time-wasting, frustration and failure — of patient and therapist alike.

Cure or Care?

One of the big decisions is whether one can aim for a 'cure' (which must be understood in relative terms) or whether only care is possible. There are several theoretical and practical issues at stake in this consideration. At one extreme are those who claim that only care is possible for brain-damaged patients; that any improvement stems only from so-called spontaneous recovery. Views range from this through various shades of opinion, which include those who feel therapy can only substitute or circumvent a deficit, those who feel that therapy can actually influence anatomical recovery and reorganisation and that underlying neuropsychological and cognitive processes can be retrained.

The divergent views are not necessarily mutually exclusive. It is likely that each of these factors operates at some stage in recovery, or is suited to some aspects of therapy but not others. Some processes might be amenable to direct retraining. Other deficits might be improved only by substituting an alternative function. Still other aspects of improvement are dependent solely on spontaneous recovery. Also, some exercises might generalise well to other behaviours, while others remain task-specific. Not only will this vary from one defect to another, but exercises will also change during the course of rehabilitation. It is likely that there are optimal times for introducing different types of therapy, and for maximising improvement in particular processes. Future research must determine these factors for dyspraxia therapy

A detailed exposition of these arguments is impossible here, but discussion can be found in Diller and Gordon (1981), Rosenthal *et al.* (1983), Rothi and Horner (1983) and Miller (1984).

In an ideal world, diagnosis would be able to pinpoint nodes of breakdown in known sensory motor processes, and therapists would be able to prescribe specific exercises that would restore or adequately circumvent the deficiency. Despite indications that this might be possible in certain cases (Weinberg, Diller, Gordon *et al.*, 1977, 1979, for examples; Miller, 1984, for summary), scholarship remains far from determining whether this will be feasible in all cases. Currently, and especially in the field of dyspraxia, exactly what underlying processes are disturbed is still far from known. One is still far from being able to offer direct intervention strategies for them.

Therapy of What? Underlying Processes

Some inkling of different varieties of disturbance is discernible from the literature. The clear instances of disconnection syndromes (Heilman, 1973; De Renzi *et al.*, 1982) would suggest therapy emphasising control through intact channels, or research devising methods of making good the disconnection. Perceptual and executive dimensions (Roy, 1981; Heilman *et al.*, 1982) will require attention in some cases. In constructional dyspraxia, especially that of non-dominant hemisphere origin, emphasis will be on visual–spatial factors. Cases of difficulty in evocation of movements (Kerschensteiner and Poeck, 1974; De Renzi *et al.*, 1982) would direct therapy towards facilitation of recall. Conceptualisation breakdown in ideational dyspraxia (Lehmkuhl and Poeck, 1981; Roy, 1983) invites development of procedures to aid overall organisation of plans. Similarly, planning disruption in pre-frontal-type dyspraxia requires therapy that will assist in the conceptualisation of the action programme; it also demands strategies that will help carry through the plan to its conclusion. Theoretically, therapy should seek techniques that aim for smoothness of flow if ideomotor dyspraxia is a problem in transition from one element of organisation to another (Kimura, 1982; Roy, 1983).

More detailed knowledge of the underlying disruptions in dyspraxia is needed before therapy based on causes rather than symptoms can be instigated. To date, most therapists have adopted a predominantly pragmatic, problem-oriented approach. They have analysed behaviour to find out when and in what ways the patient's dyspraxia presents barriers, and they documented strengths and weaknesses. Task-related therapies have been produced on the basis of these findings.

Therapy of What? Behavioural Manifestation

Before dealing with task decisions, more mention of where problems can arise will be made. It is vital to locate precisely where difficulties lie in an action. Perhaps only minimal improvement can be brought about in some instances; but, if that improvement is in a crucial element, it can alter the balance between deficiency and efficiency. It can make all the difference between a dependent, depressed individual who is unable to fit into their environment, and one who has a positive attitude and dignity, and who is in control of their life.

Identifying crucial behaviours is also vital if time is not to be wasted in directing therapy at skills or subskills which, even if (re)acquisition was successful, would not help the patient in coping with demands. An example illustrates this: a person has difficulty taking a drink of tea; undifferentiated therapy would simply involve practising drinking tea; closer examination, however, would reveal whether the person can recognise the cup, reach it properly, grasp it correctly, bring it to the mouth accurately, orient it to the mouth efficiently, control tilting, coordinate tilting with drinking, recognise errors and utilise error feedback. Once the one or more areas of breakdown have been defined more precisely, therapy can be directed more effectively and sparingly.

The types of derailment and the likely locus of their occurrence have been described for the different dyspraxias in Chapters 2 to 7. These details, plus an awareness of possible co-existing disorders or disabilities with which they might be confused, should guide observations and decision-making regarding therapy. Several case examples have been quoted already.

Therapists must also be alert to problems that may arise during therapy that can be attributable to dyspraxia. Heilman *et al*. (1975) suggest that dyspraxics (in their instance, ideomotor) have difficulties with previously learned tasks and in acquiring and retaining new material. Kimura (1977), Roy (1981) and Rothi and Heilman (1985) found similar deficits. Hence, ideomotor or other dyspraxias may be flawing performance on previously known actions and may also impair therapy in areas which involve learning new techniques, for instance, the use of lazy-tongs, long-handled shoe-horns or walking frames. New techniques required for single-handed dressing or one-handed vegetable peeling or slicing may be disrupted or thwarted by an underlying dyspraxia.

In addition, learning new movements for transfers from wheelchair to bed or toilet, or even operating a wheelchair itself, may prove difficult for dyspraxics. Previously, such patients were able to rise from a chair or position themselves on the bedside without conscious thought; the need to break down consciously the action sequence into component parts and reproduce them as a smooth sequence may be taxing precisely the area in which dyspraxic patients experience difficulty.

Therefore, a known dyspraxia must be taken into account in planning other aspects of rehabilitation; an unrecognised dyspraxia is a possible consideration in cases where expected gain fails to be achieved.

Therapeutic Techniques

Having decided that dyspraxia needs to be an area for rehabilitation, and having targeted through observation and other assessments just which behaviours require treatment, the aim will be to devise actual therapy tasks and techniques. The general principles of task design will be familiar to all therapists, and are covered in the general works cited on p. 195. These and other works also discuss issues in establishing baselines for treatment and monitoring progress. Although these matters are mentioned only in passing, it does not mean that they are any less important in dyspraxia treatment than any other field. Their inclusion in plans is taken for granted here.

Task Construction

This section deals with some central features of therapy, with specific reference to dyspraxia. Among the aims in choosing and designing tasks are to:

1. Isolated the behaviour to be rehabilitated;
2. Insure that success on the task depends on the behaviour to be trained;
3. Insure that completion does not demand performance in other areas of deficit, for example, attention, language, perception;
4. Choose task continua rather than leap from one behaviour to another unrelated one;
5. Direct continua towards a goal that will be useful in itself, or permit progress to another significant level in therapy;
6. Start intervention at the level at which the patient experiences problems;
7. Proceed in attainable steps;
8. Enable patient and therapist to monitor progress.

These points do not represent all of these needed to be considered, but are some of the central ones. The following suggestions are for areas in which to construct task continua. Suggestions for techniques to achieve the goals decided upon follow these.

Increasing Directional Complexity. Initially, movements can be in one direction and in a straight line — for example, left to right or top to bottom. This might be practised by drawing lines or moving objects or limbs. Gradually, changes in direction can be introduced: first by going back the same way, then by moving off at a right-angle and more difficult angles, leading to more complex sequences and directional changes.

Increasing the Range of Planes. To start with the above movements can be restricted to one plane, be it horizontal, diagonal or vertical. Introducing changes in plane assists transfer of movements from two- to three-dimensional space.

Varying the Sphere of Action. Changing from actions performed in personal to external space, or *vice versa*, represents a gradation in difficulty for some people.

Proximal–Distal Control. Proximally controlled gross movements will be easier than distally performed fine motor actions for most dyspraxics. Therapy can progress from predominantly proximal control to increasingly fine differentiation of distal movement.

One-Handed — Two-Handed Actions. One handed action is much easier than bi-manual co-ordination. This is especially so for dyspraxics. After a satisfactory level of one-handed control is achieved, movements of the other hand/arm (if there is no paresis) can be introduced. Proximally controlled mirror movements tend to be easiest. Static positions rather than movement is easier. This holds particularly when non-co-ordinated movements of the two limbs are introduced. For instance, the patient may be able to put both arms into the air at 45 degrees, but not to change position such that the left arm is held straight up and right arm is in front, at shoulder level. The same applies to two-handed differentiated distal actions, and in leg actions if these need to be rehabilitated (driving, dancing).

The improvement spanned by this task continuum may cover months or years of therapy, or it may never be achieved.

Number of Objects Involved. Therapy might begin with non-specific handling of a single object. Activity will involve more implements as praxic ability returns. For example, at first the person might simply be asked to hammer; later, he is asked to hammer on a particular spot; then a real nail is introduced, which has to be hit into a piece of wood. Later still, the patient is asked to fix together two pieces of wood in a set fashion. Alternatively, two-piece jig-saws can be used, that need only the sides to be placed together, rather than interlinked. Gradually, the number of pieces involved is increased. Exercises in this field can progress up to multiple-object tasks such as baking, gardening and so on.

Sophistication Needed for Objects. A hammer is easier to manage than a screwdriver, a breadknife is easier than a tin-opener. Attention must be paid to the demands individual implements place on the patient. The complexity relates to the mechanics of the implement and the task for which it is used.

These dimensions by no means exhaust the number of task continua that exist in dyspraxia rehabilitation. Other changes include: speed of presentation; speed of response required (some mild dyspraxics only break down under pressure of time); the standard of correctness demanded; the introduction of varying sizes, shapes and colours, which may be a complicating factor for constructional and pre-frontal dyspraxics especially. In addition to increases in task complexity, increased difficulty can be brought about by staged withdrawal of external supporting mechanisms.

Support Mechanisms

Again, there is no real limit to what these mechanisms might include, and methods will be found to suit individual patients. However, there are several traditional starting points.

Familiarity of Task. The more familiar and more 'automatic' the action, the easier it should be. The more familiar the environment and circumstances, the more likely the person is to succeed: hence the need to carry out therapy in realistic, conducive surroundings, particularly in the early stages. In assessment, the person may produce different performances on the ward, in the rehabilitation department's kitchen and in his own home (Smith, 1979).

Meaningfulness of Activity. The more meaningful and less abstract the action required, the higher will be the standard of response. Reinterpreting abstract, meaningless tasks in more concrete terms is a welltried therapeutic technique (see p. 209–10).

Varying Input Modality. A common practice in many therapies is to offer input through intact modalities, or through multiple channels (p. 208). Task demands can be increased both by phasing out input support and the assistance permitted from other modalities when responding. These aspects are covered in more detail later.

Amount of Information Given. As well as offering information through several modalities, the amount of data given can be varied. Someone with speech dyspraxia may be helped in recalling/realising a sound by contextualisation, for example *A, B, C, __*; or, *You sleep in a be__.* The therapist can decrease the amount of information by reducing the contextual support: *You sleep in a __*, with only mouthing of *be__*. The next step might be to exclude mouthing and say only *You sleep in a . . .*; then *You sleep . . .*; and finally, the therapist may simply use a picture of a bed or point to one to elicit the response.

The same can be achieved in manual dyspraxia by systematically removing contextual support and lead-ins. The therapist might manipulate passively the person's limb through an activity until they arrive at the sub-act in question, and then leave them to complete it alone. Alternatively, the person is allowed to carry out the act as part of an overall activity, if that helps (p. 210). The 'carrier' act must then be removed part by part until the movement in question can be produced in isolation.

Another method of aiding production by using context and then gradually withdrawing it, is to perform a movement first with a real object and then progressively without. A classic example is to encourage an oral dyspraxic to blow by holding a lighted match before the mouth. Phasing out assistance might involve: holding up a lighted and then an unlighted match; making the striking gesture but not bringing the match to the mouth; then, perhaps, after other sub-steps, simply asking the person to blow. These last strategies move away from strategies in task construction and towards the discussion of therapeutic support techniques.

Error Recognition and Utilisation

Another aspect of therapy that must be included in dyspraxia, as much as in any other behavioural therapy, is error recognition and utilisation. The detailed assessment of the individual should already have told the therapist the exact locus and type of errors. This does not guarantee that the patient recognises the errors or knows why they are involved in a particular therapeutic exercise.

This is especially so of right-hemisphere constructional dyspraxics, who have poor attention to errors. Others may recognise their errors, but fail to act upon the information; they do not utilise error feedback. This holds particularly for frontal planning dyspraxics: either they carry on indifferently, even while declaring the inadequacy of their attempts, or they pause but give up in puzzlement at how they should correct the error which they have recognised. Other patients become depressed or angry with the constant realisation that their efforts end in error, and that they cannot remedy them despite their most determined efforts. Many ideational and left-hemisphere constructional dyspraxics fall into this category.

Hence, before commencing on a task continuum, it may be necessary for the patient to be trained to recognise and appreciate precisely what is in error. Perceptual exercises of one kind or another may work in this case (p. 211).

Not traditionally recommended, but of potential use, is to have the person recognise plus or minus correct performance mimed by others. This is mentioned as it has been found helpful in some personal cases. However, the subject of pantomime recognition in brain-damaged people represents an entirely controversial issue itself (Duffy and Watkins, 1984; Heilman *et al.*, 1975; Roy, 1983). In addition, its usefulness in therapy awaits confirmation in controlled trials rather than by anecdotal reporting. However, recognising errors is only a first step. The person needs to be taught how to utilise error information to overcome difficulties (see support systems below).

Johnston and Diller (1983) report a technique for error evaluation training. Unfortunately they do not say exactly how the therapy was structured, only that before the exercise was repeated, a structured enquiry took place after each performance on how patients felt they had done.

Support Strategies

Support strategies are used to assist dyspraxics to achieve actions they would not otherwise accomplish. Again, the principles of choosing strategies will be well known to therapists. They include well recognised methods such as: input and/or output through intact channels to compensate for impaired modalities; passive manipulation; structured environment; and mechanical aids. In fact, the number and type of cues is restricted only by the therapist's ingenuity and the dyspraxic's capacity to capitalise on them.

Initially, the dyspraxic person is offered as much support as necessary to complete the action. At first, the cues will come exclusively or predominantly from the therapist; the intention is a staged withdrawal of support until total responsibility for correct performance is assumed by the patient. The dyspraxic may still be using support cues, rather than actually having re-acquired the defective underlying process, but at least they are self-initiated and not supplied by the therapist.

Two ready support strategies in dyspraxia are visual and verbal guides. Verbal support may be restricted in cases with co-existing dysphasia; the usefulness of visual support will be curtailed if visual–spatial impairment is present. This stresses the importance of differential diagnosis between language and visual–spatial factors that may be underlying such manifestations as right–left disorientation, body part naming difficulties and so on (see p. 152).

Verbal Support

At first, verbal support may be a detailed commentary by the therapist of what the patient needs to do. The detail will be determined by the nature of the task and the degree of guidance the person needs. It might be as general as 'Now take the fork; stick it in the potato; put the knife in front of the fork prongs; cut down with the knife'. Alternatively, it might have to include detailed instructions of how to grasp the fork, move it to the potato, how to stick it in and how to lift it up again, bringing the food to the mouth.

Gradually, instructions are made less specific. The dyspraxic takes over self-direction either by learning the instructions or by having them in written form to refer to — initially constantly and then intermittently, first with full details and then with key words only.

It should not be assumed that verbalisation by itself will work like a magic wand, even for those who can benefit from it. The person will most likely have to be taught how to follow directions, and other motor and visual teaching may be needed to perfect sub-parts of the action. Verbal support is envisaged as a means of providing an external structure for behaviour that cannot be managed effectively within its own sphere. Verbalisation does not replace planning, but supports it. Instructions should be clear, unambiguous and geared to the problems the person experiences. Therapists must experiment to see whether verbalisation before or during the act, or both, assists better.

Verbal support is potentially most helpful in constructional dyspraxia of non-dominant hemisphere origin, in problems of visual scanning (Stanton, Yorkston, Kenyon and Beukelman, 1981) or visual–spatial synthesis. It can be used to remind the person beforehand which features need to be entered into a diagram, and to express the spatial relationships the parts must have to each other while drawing the diagram. The same strategy could be used in dressing to help gain the correct order for putting on clothes, and for monitoring which parts relate to which body parts while dressing.

Labels attached to the clothes can assist. Sleeves can be labelled 'right arm' or 'left arm', jumpers can have tags denoting 'front', 'back', 'top' and 'bottom'. Shoes can have directions for 'right', 'left', 'heel' and 'toe'. More explicit instructions could include 'This bit over head' or 'Pull up to shoulder'.

The same strategies can be exploited in ideational and dominant hemisphere constructional dyspraxia, where language ability permits. Directions should be suited to individual cases. Therapists should not expect the same labels and instructions to be applicable to different disorders. In ideational dyspraxia, the aim will be to aid the conceptualisation of the overall plan and the correct sequence of moves, as much as improving the spatial organisation, which will be a more prominent feature in constructional dyspraxia.

Luria (1948, translation 1963) introduced many examples in which verbalisation helped to overcome perseveratory responses, initiation difficulties and forward-planning problems in frontal-type dyspraxia. For instance, in trying to maintain particular rhythms of movements, phrases were found with stress patterns that supplied the rhythm. A circle and a square were difficult to draw for one man, but as soon as he verbalised these as 'sun' and 'house', he was able to draw them freely. Another man struggled to draw the abstract sequence

$$\equiv \;\Big|\; \underline{\quad}$$

but succeeded when they could be verbalised as a 'railway', 'barrier' and 'country road'.

Not everything can be put into words, and that is a limiting factor for verbalisation. Gazzaniga (1978) cites the example of someone who apparently improved on block-design, but still failed on a wire figures test. It transpired that the individual had developed a verbal support strategy for himself: it worked for the blocks, but not for the wire.

Visual Support

Several different approaches can be described: pictorial support; visual landmarks; coding systems and environmental manipulation.

Pictorial Aids. These have been employed to accompany an entire action sequence or to illustrate key moves in a particular task. Thus the graphics for making a coin-box phone-call might include: lifting the receiver; resting coin in slot; dialling; pressing coin in slot.

For dressing, the sheet or series of cards might include: clothes laid out in order; putting left leg into pants; putting right leg into pants; pulling pants up to waist; and so on.

These examples represent relatively non-specific instructions. More detailed guidance may be necessary for some patients, or at particular junctures in certain actions for people otherwise able to cope. Someone might be able to chop off the top of a boiled egg, but be unable to get the spoon in to eat it. Pictures could show: how to steady the egg with one hand (provided the patient is not hemiplegic); the angle at which to put the spoon in; how to get the egg on to it; and how to lift it out again without dropping it.

Direct graphic representation, in personal experience, is suitable for overall organisation but becomes difficult when minutiae or complex relationships have to be represented.

Landmarks and coding systems better suit such cases. As with verbal aids, it should not be assumed that performance will improve just because guidelines are used. The patient will have to be taught how to exploit them. The hope is that learning through their use will be considerably more easy and bring about improvement more quickly than concentrating directly on the dyspraxic weakness.

Landmark Techniques. One technique familiar to most people who have learnt to write is the use of horizontal lines to define the space within which an action should be carried out (Figure 8.1).

Figure 8.1: Use of Horizontal Lines to Define Writing Space

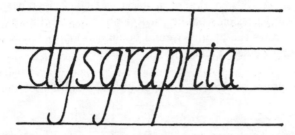

Elaborations of this system may assist letter spacing. For example, a particular feature at the left-hand margin can help directionality and scanning; numbered lines can assist downward progression (Weinberg *et al.*, 1977) (Figure 8.2).

Figure 8.2: Left-Hand Margin Feature and Numbered Lines

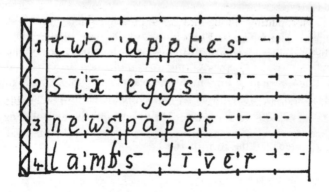

One patient of Luria (1948, translated 1963) failed to produce the sequence

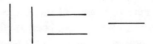

but succeeded when the outline

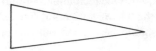

was introduced.

Landmarks can also be drawn on objects to facilitate their use. Matching shapes or letters on separate parts can help in object assembly, for example, arrows can be drawn on a bottle and top to enable them to be put back together (Figure 8.3).

Figure 8.3: Arrows on Bottle and Top to Enable Their Alignment

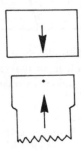

Arrows can be used for directionality. Luria's colleagues (Luria, 1948, translated 1963) used arrows and lines for the angle or arc of movement to guide hammering and sawing. The same technique has been adopted for cutting bread and opening tins. A combination of verbal and visual support has been used for a man who had trouble unlocking doors. The word 'Lock' was the guide, and the following signs helped him to use a key: L represented the angle at which to put the key in;

◯ signalled the turn of the key;

C meant the return.

Colour Coding. This provides a productive system of landmarks, especially for patients with poor language and/or poor spatial perception who have difficulty matching shapes. For example, matching colours might have been used instead of the two arrows on the bottle top.

Colour coding permits extension beyond single part-to-part matching, by the setting up of complex sequences. Dressing can be helped in this way. Different colours can represent left, right, top, bottom, back and front. The order of putting on clothes and orientation of clothes to body parts can be improved using a master card which sets out the order in which colours are to be tackled.

For instance, the master card at one stage may show the progression red-blue, where red is 'left', blue is 'sock'. This is followed by blue-green, where green is 'inside of trouser leg'; then comes yellow-black, where yellow is 'top of trousers', black the 'waist'. The patient matches the colours shown until dressing is complete. The colour sequences could just as easily relate to getting a cup of coffee, folding a letter into an envelope, putting money in a gas or electric meter, or whatever the person's problem is.

Environmental Structuring. This is especially important for patients who have difficulty in manipulating their environment. The number of implements a person can mix up can be reduced simply by conducting therapy in an uncluttered environment. This can be encouraged outside the clinic, too. The objects used should be as straightforward as possible, without having any unusual shapes, attachments, frills or novel (to the patient) ways of operation. Lighting should not throw any confusing shadows. Patterns on clothes or utensils should be avoided if they only add to the likelihood of derailment.

Gadgets and furniture that are simple to operate may be advisable in cases where it is going to make the difference between freedom and dependency. For example, an electric cooker may be easier to operate than gas; an automatic car may be easier than one with manual gears; a push-button hi-fi may be easier than a dial-controlled one; making a cup of instant coffee is easier than percolated or filter coffee; slip-on shoes and elasticated trousers will be easier than laces, straps and buckles.

Guided Imagery

The use of verbal, visual and motor images has been used extensively in other fields of brain-damage rehabilitation, particularly for memory problems. The idea is that the person uses a verbal, visual or action image which they can remember and picture mentally in order to cue them into something that cannot be remembered. It is particularly useful where part of a disorder is a difficulty in evocation or initiation of activities.

The example on p. 110 of using the more automatic and better retained *Friday* to tune into *fried egg* is an example of verbal-guided imagery helping the speech dyspraxic. Complex patterns can be developed by using successions of words. One patient used a variation of melodic intonation therapy (p. 111) to remember and to say where he lived. He could not say 'Carrickfergus' in isolation, but could if he first hummed the song 'I wish I were in Carrickfergus'.

The example on p. 205 in which the drawing of circles and squares is helped by imagining them to be the sun and a house could be interpreted as an example of visual-guided imagery. Visualising a train signal or crane, where these are familiar to the subject, can help in arm movements and postures, or in forming letter shapes.

Action initiation can be assisted by finding a more automatic eliciting image than the one demanded by the task in hand. Stretching out the arm directly in front for whatever reason may be done hesitantly, if at all; but when the patient is asked to imagine he is punching someone, the movement might be produced instantly. The therapist should remember to duck. The dyspraxic may be unable to draw a circular shape or produce a circular motion as needed when dialling the telephone or getting ice cream out of the dish, and so on. If the patient can produce the action spontaneously for stirring tea, then it could be exploited for recalling and initiating these similar other movements.

As with verbal and visual imagery, multiple sequences can be built up to assist more complex actions. The only restriction is the number of reliable associations that can be uncovered for the individual, and their ability to use them.

Aids

In general, the usual range of dressing, walking and other daily living aids that might assist non-dyspraxic, stroke or other brain-damaged patients, do not significantly help dyspraxics. In fact, they often introduce a complicating factor (see p. 199) if the aid requires the introduction of motor learning and unfamiliar tasks. Where improvement is found with aids, it can usually be put down to better performance regarding one of the non-dyspraxic disabilities. When an aid is sufficiently close to a previous behaviour but simplifies it, then it may prove beneficial, for example, the use of press studs instead of buttons, or nail clippers instead of scissors.

Computers have been hailed as a great step forward for therapeutic possibilities. However, optimism must be more guarded regarding dyspraxia therapy. In certain respects, they do offer advantages: the variety of programmes that can be used; the possibility of adapting them to the individual's deficits; the capacity for storage and recall of past performance; the opportunity for the patient to work independently and at their own speed; the scope offered for making therapy attractive to poorly motivated patients. But against these potential gains, one has to weigh up the fact that computer technology is a novel area to most people; it requires the learning and operation of new motor programmes, which is precisely the area of difficulty for dyspraxics. Given the variety of problems presented by them, the number and variations of programmes required will be considerable.

One could envisage using computers to give direct visual and verbal support and feedback for a number of manual tasks performed at the keyboard or joystick. Problems of rhythm and switching of motor programmes, one- and two-handed co-ordination, hand–eye co-ordination, tracking, speed of reaction and motor decision-making all suggest themselves as good candidates. The graphic display capacity would seem well suited for those patients who have a visual–spatial perceptual deficit as part of their disability.

Hi-tech approaches to therapy will expand the options available to therapists if programmes are geared directly to the dyspraxic's difficulties (as opposed to off-the-shelf, general, perceptual or motor software) and are applied at the right time — provided the introduction of the computer does not mean added problems. Therapists should take up the challenge of capitalising on the potential offered by computers: but they are not, and will not become, a panacea.

Perceptual Training

One area that many will feel warrants close attention in dyspraxia is perceptual training, which has not been a prime focus of this chapter. While some dyspraxics show perceptual disabilities (Roy, 1981; Heilman *et al.*, 1982), others perform normally on perceptual tasks (Deutsch, 1984b). The only patients consistently showing perceptual defects are those with non-dominant hemisphere constructional dyspraxia — which is essentially a visual–spatial disorder in any case. Thus, while perceptual deficits must be sought in assessment, they are not expected in all dyspraxics.

Advocacy of a blanket application of perceptual therapy in dyspraxia is based on the influence of certain works on developmental dyspraxia (for example, Ayres, 1973, 1979). While there are strong arguments for such an approach with children, it is less clear whether, or how, perceptual deficits directly affect motor performance in adults. The finding of normal praxis in some perceptually disordered patients, or normal perception in many dyspraxics and continued dyspraxia in patients where a perceptual disturbance has ameliorated or disappeared, all question the urgency of perceptual therapy in dyspraxia. There are no straight answers to the issue, which must be resolved by further research.

Another reason for not concentrating on perceptual input has been a desire to alter the current imbalance in detailing therapy for motor aspects of dyspraxia. Perceptual therapy has been amply reported elsewhere (Siev and Freishtat, 1976; Weinberg *et al.*, 1979; Young, Collins and Hren, 1983), as well as the general textbooks of different disciplines quoted above (p. 195).

Counselling

Part of the rehabilitation team's role will be to counsel patient and family and, where necessary, friends and employers. Clearly, the subject of discussion will be the implications of the cerebral trauma for the entire personal and family life. The following remarks are confined to the more direct effects of dyspraxia.

Dyspraxia gradually creeps up on most people: it does not leap out like a physical deformity; it cannot be seen or experienced like a hemiplegia or an epileptic attack; it cannot be heard like a dysphasia or dysarthria; it cannot even be sensed or explained in the same way that primary sensory loss, visual field defects or ataxia can. Yet it penetrates into the individual's most private life. It catches them at the most unsuspecting moments and throws them down in bewilderment, embarrassment, shame and anger. It invites wrath from usually under-standing partners or hollow words of comfort: 'It'll be all right.'

But it is not all right. The person can see that his limbs have full mobil-ity: 'The doctor said my reflexes were fine; the physiotherapist said my strength was good; the feeling has come back to my arm; and I can recognise people and places now, and what things are. Yet I fail to get in the door, cannot fix the washer on the tap, or the light-bulb as I used to.'

In hospital the disability could be rationalised away as being part of the general upset. This idea may have been encouraged by well-meaning but unsuspecting medical staff. It is easy to explain away the clumsiness as the consequence of a hemiplegia.

These are the views and feelings with which a counsellor will have to deal. On the one hand, the patient is apparently able-bodied or has recognisable disability; but on the other hand he continually fails in actions that they ought to be able to manage. In turn, this usually leads to cer-tain reactions from sufferer and associates.

Dyspraxia is one of the sequelae of brain damage that is most easy to miss and misinterpret. Health-care workers and family can be misled into branding dyspraxics as confused, disoriented, demented, subnormal or hysterical — thereby condemning them to the most unjust treatment.

Differential diagnosis should exclude these factors, or establish their degree of co-occurrence; and people who have contact with the patient should then be counselled accordingly.

They need to understand what activities may be affected, and in what ways and why. They must be shown the ways in which the person can be assisted and what his true capabilities are. In one personal case, the patient's sister was reported by nursing staff never to speak to her sister when she visited. When asked about this, the healthy sister told how she had first tried to get her sister to say things, but only got non-specific sounds and gestures as a reply. She had tried to get her to write, but had argued with her sister for writing in scrawly capitals instead of normal script, so she had not tried again, accepting that she had become a baby. When she was shown how to elicit speech from her sister and it was suggested she look at *what* instead of *how* her sister was writing, she was astounded at her capability.

The same explanations and reassurance should be given to dyspraxic patients themselves. In cases of accompanying dysphasia it is doubly important and reassuring that therapists should verbalise the patient's fears, frustrations and despair about the action disability.

Another set of labels frequently unjustifiably hung on dyspraxics is that they are inattentive, apathetic, indifferent, obstinate, irritable and lazy. These traits may also be consequences of brain damage and interact with the dyspraxic condition. Where they are secondary to the dyspraxia, they can be improved through the attitude the people have towards themselves and through the attitudes of others, providing everyone appreciates what dyspraxia means. Timely counselling can prevent these features arising as secondary symptoms.

Follow-ups of head injuries (Jennet and Teasdale, 1981; Bond, 1983; Thomsen, 1984) suggest that, initially, the individual's and family's main concerns are the preservation of life; later the main physical disabilities, and in the long-term, the psychosocial sequelae are of more concern. Personality changes are a possibility after brain lesion. It is always worth checking for an unrecognised dyspraxia as a source of intra- and interpersonal conflict in treating these longer-term consequences.

These remarks give only the briefest glimpse at the position of counselling in dyspraxia rehabilitation. The central points are that: it must happen; the counselling must be consistent and co-ordinated if coming from several sources; and the aloofness of the therapist and mystique about the disorder should not become added features of that disorder.

Therapy — An Example

While tasks, techniques and strategies have been outlined separately, most people will be using input from several directions at any one time, or switch from one strategy to another as therapy progresses. Writing therapy illustrates this well. It might start with strong visual guidance; for example, tracking directly over single, motorically simple, block capital letters. Even this might prove too difficult for some. Initial intervention for these patients, provided they can recognise letters and other shapes, may also require active hand guidance by the therapist or the use of a template. Further support may involve verbalisation of the strokes to be made and their direction. At first, the therapist will have provided the commentary, but with the intention that it should be taken over by the patient. Alternatively or additionally, arrows, numbers and colours may be used to denote the order and direction of strokes.

Imagery may play a part. Remembering letters in terms of familiar objects is one example — A as the Eiffel or Blackpool Tower; H as Gaelic or rugby football posts; O as a ball. Later on, patients may be able to produce a letter with which they have difficulty, by tackling it with reference to letters they can manage. S can be seen as $c + $ ɔ; h as $l + n$; y as $u + j$.

Once tracing whole letters, connecting dots, direct copying and use of landmarks has been phased out, directionality may become a larger problem. A whole page landmark (Figure 8.2) or verbalisation may assist — for example, 'Good side to bad side', or *vice versa*, if the person is hemiplegic, and head-foot for top-bottom.

For some individuals, successful writing may be only the icing on the cake following lengthy therapy involving proximal, whole-arm movements and months of increasingly fine differentiation. Therapy on achieving a workable grasp may have had to precede writing proper.

Differential diagnosis must have decided whether the dysgraphia is due to visual–perceptual, motor recall, motor execution or whatever dysfunction within the range of visual–motor dysgraphias (see Hécaen and Albert, 1978; Benson, 1979; Roeltgen, 1985); it must also have assessed for an underlying language disorder. It should be recalled that, in lesions of transcallosal fibres, there are different types of writing disorder according to stimulus mode and which hand is used (Ch. 6).

Brown *et al.* (1983) describe an interesting method of exploiting the phenomenon of 'hemiplegic writing'. In these cases with aphasia, the person is unable to write with the left hand, but shows some ability to write to dictation and name objects held in the left hand if the right arm can be mobilised. Using a penholder and skateboard prosthesis, Brown *et al.* exploited the preserved shoulder joint movement to enable patients who demonstrate this picture to write.

Following the principle of tapping more automatic control, some words might be produced by otherwise agraphic people. Such productions are nearly always made in the person's accustomed handwriting rather than in block capitals. Name, address and familiar objects might all be named in writing this way. Typically, performance is better if the person does not actually concentrate on the writing aspect. Analogous to the use of more automatic utterances as carrier phrases or lead-ins in speech, these residual skills can do the same for writing.

Conclusion

It is not suggested that these procedures are going to suit each and every dyspraxic patient and their particular picture of disability. They are presented as instances that, from personal experience, have seemed to work for certain individuals with certain problems. Neither is it claimed that the procedures involved are what actually brought about any improvement, or that, even if they were responsible, it was for the reasons one would imagine.

The aim in this chapter is to concentrate on more central needs in rehabilitation which have hitherto been neglected. The chapter has ignored more general aspects of management such as principles in choosing and designing tasks. It is hoped that the detailed chapters on assessment and other works referred to that deal with overall management of neurologically impaired people will have provided this background. Neither has it dealt with the way in which dyspraxia therapy might fit in with other therapies (physical, language, perceptual, social). It is assumed that these are matters of general management, as is deciding who will be responsible for the various aspects of therapy and the treatment time-scale. There are no specific answers to these questions; each new case will pose its own new set of queries.

The overall attitude adopted by this chapter has been pragmatic — that the aim of therapy is to restore peoples ability to look after themselves and function as a member of the community, rather than to train them to pass the bi-dimensional, multichromatic linear object abstract projection sub-test (in other words, the 2-D coloured stick design) in Joe Soap's psycho-cerebro-socio-cognitive-neuro-rehabilitational battery. However, there is some indication that there may be some generalisation from more abstract therapy to more concrete activities (see p. 195, 207); in an ideal world, such exercises would be prescribed to remediate the dysfunctions underlying diverse difficulties. Unfortunately, this is not such a world and it is the task of research to set us on the road. In the meantime, a more practically guided approach must continue to be used.

In choosing task continua, it has been emphasised that defining the crucial behaviour to be trained is decisive. The steps in the continuum should be within the bounds of learnability, and the end-product should be something that the person will be able to make effective use of, and that will produce a desirable change in capabilities. Furthermore, the technique itself must not become the end of therapy: just because a person shows a certain behaviour, should not mean that a particular technique is applied automatically without regard to whether, when or how such therapy will be of use to the individual.

The suggestions in this chapter are offered as starting points for therapists to explore avenues which might help their own dyspraxic patients. More importantly in the long run, the intervention possibilities described could serve as starting points for properly controlled studies, if dyspraxia therapy is to be placed on a more scientific basis. These studies should investigate whether or not the strategies really are effective in terms of bringing about improvement, and find which techniques are best applicable to which types of disorder, and at which stages of rehabilitation.

Another research aim should be to determine which strategies produce generalised advance and which ones appear restricted to bringing about improvement in only one behaviour. Until these research aims have been fulfilled, dyspraxia therapy — however well delivered — will remain on an *ad hoc* basis with only anecdotal support for its efficacy. Controlled clinical trials are paramount to bring therapy out of this state, to improve therapists' accountability and expertise in choosing strategies and monitoring progress and, of course, the primary aim — to offer the dyspraxic person worthwhile intervention.

Finally, through all the research and striving to understand the physiology, neurology, psychology and sociology of dyspraxia, throughout all endeavours to perfect quantitative, qualitative and observational assessments, and throughout all the searching and clinical testing of the whole range of therapeutic measures devised, it must be remembered that dyspraxia is a disorder suffered by human beings with souls, feelings, hopes and fears. They must not be failed.

> The average person will never understand the extent of my illness, never know what it's like unless he experiences it himself.

L. Zasetsky (Luria, 1972, p. 129)

GLOSSARY

Agnosia: Loss of ability to recognise sensory stimuli (principally visual, auditory or tactile), despite intact primary senses.

Allophones: Subdivisions of a phoneme (q.v.). The two different /k/ sounds in *k*eel and *c*oal are allophones of the phoneme /k/.

Amnestic Dysphasia: see anomic.

Anomic Dysphasia: Language disturbance where the principal problem lies in retrieving/recalling words.

Anosognosia: Denial, non-recognition of, or indifference of patients to their disability.

Astereognosia: Inability to recognise objects by touch, despite intact primary sensation.

Broca's Dysphasia: Language disturbance characterised by telegram-like utterances, lacking formal grammatical structure and containing mainly nouns and verbs. Relatively good comprehension.

Conduction Dysphasia: See Chapter 4.

Dysgnosia: Less severe agnosia (q.v.); faulty recognition.

Dysgraphia: Disorder of writing.

Dyslexia: Disorder of reading.

Dysphasia: Disorder of language.

Euclidean Space: Geometrical, three-dimensional space.

Fluent Dysphasia: Language disturbance in which the natural flow and intonation of speech remain essentially intact (cf. conduction; non-fluent; Wernicke's).

Global Dysphasia: Language disturbance severely affecting all areas of language functioning.

Gnosis: Recognition, perception. See agnosia, dysgnosia.

Haptic: Referring to the science of touch, or all the factors (tactile, proprioceptive, kinaesthetic and so on) contributing to the sense of contact.

Jargon Dysphasia: Language disturbance in which, for one reason or another, the utterance is incomprehensible to the listener, though not necessarily to the speaker.

Morphology: In linguistics, the study of word modification — talk-talked; foot-feet; well-unwell, etc. In traditional terms, accidence or inflection.

Microgeny: In this book, the details of the origins and development of

217

individual actions (cf. ontogeny, phylogeny).

Non-fluent Dysphasia: Language disturbance in which the natural flow and intonation of speech are halting, hesitant, disrupted (cf. fluent, Broca's, transcortical motor).

Optokinetic Nystagmus: Nystagmus induced by looking at a moving object.

Ontogeny: Development of the individual (person or animal) (cf. microgeny, phylogeny).

Paraphasia: Production of inappropriate sounds, syllables, words, phrases, in trying to speak. Severe paraphasia may lead to jargon (q.v.).

Parapraxia: Production of inappropriate movements, or part movements, in trying to carry out actions (cf. Chapter 2).

Phoneme: Minimum division of sound, that is considered by speakers of a language to constitute a contrast with other sounds. A phoneme is actually a collective label for several different sounds which nevertheless are heard as being identical by speakers of the language — for example, the /p/ sounds in *pie*, *spy*, *halfpenny* are all pronounced differently, yet are all heard as the phoneme /p/ by English speakers; *pie-buy* contrasts the phonemes /p/ and /b/ (cf. allophone).

Phonetics: Science of the detailed description of speech sounds according to their articulatory and acoustic properties.

Phonology: Study of linguistic sound systems.

Phylogeny: Development of the species (cf. microgeny, ontogeny).

Pursuit Movements: Smooth tracking movements (of the eyes).

Saccadic Movements: Quick darting, saltatory movements (of the eyes).

Semantics: Referring to meaning systems.

Sensory Extinction: Non-perception of one stimulus (visual, auditory, or tactile) when two stimuli are presented simultaneously via the one modality.

Syntax: The structure of language. In traditional terms, grammar.

Topographical Space: Space as related to specific landmarks of an object or environment, or between features of these.

Transcortical-Motor Dysphasia: Language disturbance with good repetition skills: poor or absent spontaneous speech; difficulty in initiation of utterances, but once initiated well pronounced. Comprehension relatively well spared.

Vestibulo-Ocular Reflex: Maintains visual stability during head movement; seen as a rotation of the eyes in the opposite direction when the head is quickly turned.

Wernicke's Dysphasia: Language disturbance characterised by fluent (q.v.) utterances which, however, contain various types of paraphasias (q.v) to varying degrees. With grammatical errors, they can make utterances poorly intelligible. Wernicke's dysphasics have relatively poor comprehension.

BIBLIOGRAPHY

Abercrombie, M. (1964) *Perceptual and Visuo-Motor Disorders in Cerebral Palsy*, Heinemann, London

Agostoni, E., Coletti, A., Orlando, G. and Tredici, G. (1983) 'Apraxia in Deep Cerebral Lesions', *J. Neurol. Neurosurg. Psychiat.*, *46*, 804–08

Akelaitis, A. (1944–45) 'Studies on the Corpus Callosum, IV: Diagnostic Dyspraxia in Epileptics Following Partial and Complete Section of the Corpus Callosum', *Am. J. Psychiat.*, *101*, 594–99

Araie, M., Ozawa, T. and Awaya, Y. (1977) 'A Case of Congenital Ocular Motor Apraxia with Cerebellospinal Degeneration', *Jpn. J. Ophthalmol.*, *21*, 355

Aram, D. and Nation, J. (1982) *Child Language Disorders*, Mosby, St Louis

Archer, L. (1977) 'Blissymbolics — a Nonverbal Communication System', *J. Speech Hear. Dis.*, *42*, 4, 568–79

Arena, R. and Gainotti, G. (1978) 'Constructional Apraxia and Visuoperceptive Disabilities in Relation to Laterality of Cerebral Lesions', *Cortex, 14*, 4, 463–73

Arnheim, D. and Sinclair, W. (1975) *The Clumsy Child. A Program of Motor Therapy*, Mosby, St Louis

Arrigoni, G. and De Renzi, E. (1964) 'Constructional Apraxia and Hemispheric Locus of Lesion', *Cortex, 1*, 170–97

Arthuis, M. (1968) 'L'Ataxie-Télangiectasie', *La Médicine Infantile, 3*, 213–30

Assal, G. and Regli, P. (1980) 'Syndrome de Disconnexion Visuo-Verbale et Visuo-Gestuelle', *Rev. Neurol. (Paris), 136*, 5, 365–76

Auerbach, S. and Alexander, M. (1981) 'Pure Agraphia and Unilateral Optic Ataxia Associated with a Left Superior Parietal Lobe Lesion', *J. Neurol. Neurosurg. Psychiat.*, *44*, 430–32

Ayres, A. (1973) *Sensory Integration and Learning Disorders*, Western Psychol. Services, Los Angeles

———— (1979) *Sensory Integration and the Child*, Western Psychol. Services, Los Angeles

———— (1980) *Southern California Sensory Integration Tests Manual — Revised*, Western Psychol. Services, Los Angeles

Badian, N. (1983) 'Dyscalculia and Nonverbal Disorders of Learning' in H. Myklebust (ed.), *Progress in Learning Disabilities*, Grune & Stratton, New York

Baker, J. (1981) 'A Psycho-motor Approach to the Assessment and Treatment of Clumsy Children', *Physiotherapy, 67*, 12, 356–63

Baloh, R., Yee, R. and Boder, E. (1977) 'Eye Movements in Ataxia Telangiectasia', *Neurol.*, *28*, 1099–1104

Barbizet, J., Degos, J-D., Duizabo, P. and Chartier B. (1974) 'Syndrome de Déconnection Interhémisphérique d'Origine Ischémique', *Rev. Neurol. (Paris), 130*, 3–4, 127–41

————, Degos, J., Lejeune, A. and LeRoy, A. (1978) 'Syndrome de Dysconnection Inter-Hémisphérique avec Dyspraxie Diagnostique au Cours d'une Maladie de Marchiafava-Bignami', *Rev. Neurol. (Paris), 134*, 12, 781–89

Basso, A., Luzzatti, C. and Spinnler, H. (1980) 'Is Ideomotor Apraxia the Outcome of Damage to Well-defined Regions of the Left Hemisphere?', *J. Neurol. Neurosurg. Psychiat.*, *43*, 118–26

Baum, B. and Hall, K. (1981) 'Relationship Between Constructional Praxis and Dressing in the Head-injured Adult', *Am. J. Occup. Ther.*, *35*, 7, 438–42

Benson, D. (1979) *Aphasia, Alexia and Agraphia*, Churchill, Edinburgh

————, Cummings, J. and Tsai, S. (1982) 'Angular Gyrus Syndrome Simulating Alzheimer's Disease', *Arch. Neurol.*, *39*, Oct., 616–20

220

Benton, A. (1961) 'Fiction of the 'Gerstmann Syndrome' ', *J. Neurol. Neurosurg. Psychiat.*, 24, 176–81
────── (1974) *Revised Visual Retention Test*, Psychol. Corporation, New York
────── and Fogel, M. (1962) 'Three-dimensional Constructional Praxis', *Arch. Neurol.*, 7, 347–54
Ben-Yishay, Y., Diller, L., Gerstman, L. and Haas, A. (1968) 'Relationship Between Impersistence, Intellectual Function and Outcome of Rehabilitation in Patients with Left Hemiplegia', *Neurology, (Minneap.)*, 18, 852–61
Bergès, J. and Lézine, I. (1963, transl. 1965) *The Imitation of Gestures*, Heinemann, London
Black, F.W. and Bernard, B. (1984) 'Constructional Apraxia as a Function of Lesion Locus and Size in Patients with Focal Brain Damage', *Cortex, 20*, 1, 111–20
────── and Strub, R. (1976) 'Constructional Apraxia in Patients with Discrete Missile Wounds of the Brain', *Cortex, 12*, 3, 212–20
Blumstein, S. (1973) *A Phonological Investigation of Aphasic Speech*, Mouton, Hague
Bogen, J. (1969) 'The Other Side of the Brain 1: Dysgraphia and Dyscopia Following Cerebral Commissurotomy', *Bull. L. Angeles Neurol. Soc., 34*, 2, 73–105
────── (1985) 'The Callosal Syndromes' in K. Heilman and E. Valenstein (eds), *Clinical Neuropsychology*, 2nd edn, Oxford University Press, Oxford
Boll, T. (1981) 'The Halstead-Reitan Neuropsychology Battery' in S. Filskov and T. Boll (eds), *Handbook of Clinical Neuropsychology*, Wiley, New York
Boller, F., Passafiume, D., Keefe, N., Rogers, K., Morrow, L. and Kim, Y. (1984) 'Visuospatial Impairment in Parkinson's Disease', *Arch. Neurol., 41*, 5, 485–90
Bond, M. (1983) 'Effects on the Family System' in M. Rosenthal *et al.* (eds), *Rehabilitation of the Head-Injured Adult*, Davis, Philadelphia
Borden, G. (1979) 'Interpretation of Research on Feedback Interruption in Speech', *Brain, Lang.*, 7, 307–19
Botez, M. (1979) 'Optic Ataxia and Apraxia of Gaze' (letter to ed.), *Neurology, 29*, 1319–20
Bower, T. (1977) *The Perceptual World of the Child*, Fontana/Open Books, Glasgow
Bowman, C., Hodson, B. and Simpson, R. (1980) 'Oral Apraxia and Aphasic Misarticulations' in R. Brookshire (ed.), *Clinical Aphasiology, Conference Proceedings*, BRK, Minneapolis
Bradley, L. (1983) 'Organisation of Visual, Phonological and Motor Strategies' in 'Learning to Read and to Spell', in U. Kirk (ed.), *Neuropsychology of Language, Reading and Spelling*, Academic Press, New York
Brion, S. and Jedynak, C-P. (1972) 'Troubles du Transfert Interhémisphérique. A Propos de Trois Observations de Tumeurs du Corps Calleux. Le Signe de la Main Étrangère', *Rev. Neurol. (Paris), 126*, 4, 257–66
────── and Jedynak, C-P. (1975) *Les Troubles du Transfert Interhémisphérique*, Masson, Paris
Brown, J. (1972) *Aphasia, Apraxia, Agnosia*, Thomas, Springfield, Illinois
────── (1977) *Mind, Brain, Consciousness*, Academic Press, New York
────── (1983) 'Emergence and Time in Microgenetic Theory', *J. Amer. Acad. Psychoanalysis, 11*, 1, 35–54
──────, Leader, B. and Blum, C. (1983) 'Hemiplegic Writing in Severe Aphasia', *Brain Lang., 10*, 204–15
Bruininks, R. (1978) *Bruininks-Osersetsky Test of Motor Proficiency*, NFER, Windsor
Buckingham, H. (1979) 'Explanation in Apraxia with Consequences for the Concept of Apraxia of Speech' *Brain Lang., 8*, 202–26
────── (1983) 'Apraxia of Language v. Apraxia of Speech' in R. McGill (ed.), *Memory and Control of Actions*, North Holland, Amsterdam
Burr, L. (1979) 'Treatment of the Child with Dyspraxia', *Brit. J. Occup. Therapy, 42*, 2, 34–39
────── (1984) 'Perceptual Motor Disorders' in S. Levitt (ed.), *Paediatric Developmental Therapy*, Blackwell, Oxford

Cahn, L. and Hodges, J. (1974) 'Cognitive–Perceptual-Motor Dysfunction and Occupational Therapy', *Academic Therapy*, *9*, 5, 335–48
Cambier, J., Elghozi, D. and Strube, E. (1980) 'Lésions du Thalamus Droit avec Syndrome de l'Hémisphère Mineur. Discussion du Concept de Négligence Thalamique', *Rev. Neurol. (Paris)*, *136*, 2, 105–16
———, Graveleau, P., Decroix, K., Elghozi, D. and Masson, M. (1983) 'Le Syndrome de l'Artère Choroidienne Antérieure. Étude Neuropsychologique de 4 Cas', *Rev. Neurol. (Paris)*, *139*, 10, 553–59
Carecchi, A. and Gainotti, G. (1977) 'Forme Congenite ed Acquisite della Cosiddetta 'Aprassia Oculo-Motoria' ', *Acta Neurol. (Napoli)*, *32*, 5, 645–53
Carr, J. and Shepherd, R. (1980) *Physiotherapy in Disorders of the Brain*, Heinemann, London
Cermak, S. (1985) 'Developmental Dyspraxia' in E. Roy (ed.), *Neuropsychological Studies of Apraxia and Related Disorders*, Elsevier, Amsterdam
———, Coster, W. and Drake, C. (1980) 'Representational and Nonrepresentational Gestures in Boys with Learning Disabilities', *Am. J. Occup. Therapy*, *34*, 1, 19–26
Christensen, A-L. (1975) *Luria's Neuropsychological Investigation Manual*, Munksgaard, Copenhagen
CIBA Foundation Symposium (1984) *Functions of the Basal Ganglia*, Symposium 107, Pitman, London
Cicci, R. (1983) 'Disorders of Written Langauge' in H. Myklebust (ed.), *Progress in Learning Disabilities*, Grune, New York
Cogan, D. (1952) 'A Type of Congenital Ocular Motor Apraxia Presenting Jerky Head Movements', *Trans. Amer. Acad. of Ophthalmology*, *56*, 853–62
——— (1966) 'Congenital Ocular Motor Apraxia', *Canad. J. Ophthal.*, *1*, 253–60
——— and Adams, R. (1953) 'A Type of Paralysis of Conjugate Gaze (Ocular Motor Apraxia)', *Arch. Ophthalmol.*, *50*, 434–42
———, Chu, F., Reingold, D. and Tychsen, L. (1980) 'A Long-term Follow-up of Congenital Ocular Motor Apraxia, Case Report', *Neuro-ophthalmol.*, *1*, 2, 145–7
———, Chu, F.C., Reingold, D. and Barranger, J. (1981) 'Ocular Motor Signs in some Metabolic Diseases', *Arch. Ophthalmol.*, *99*, 1802–8
Conrad, K., Cermak, S. and Drake, C. (1983) 'Differentiation of Praxis among Children', *Am. J. Occup. Therapy*, *37*, 7, 466–73
Consoli, S. (1979) 'Étude des Strategies Constructives Secondaires aux Lésions Hémisphériques', *Neuropsychologia*, *17*, 3–4, 303–13
Dabul, B. (1979) *Apraxia Battery for Adults*, C.C. Public, Tigard, Oregon
——— and Bollier, B. (1976) 'Therapeutic Approaches to Apraxia', *J. Speech Hear. Dis.*, *41*, 268–76
Damasio, A. (1985) 'The Frontal Lobes' in K. Heilman and E. Valenstein (eds), *Clinical Neuropsychology*, 2nd edn, Oxford University Press, Oxford
——— and Benton, A. (1979) 'Impairment of Hand Movements under Visual Guidance', *Neurology (Minneap.)*, *29*, 170–8
Damasio, H. and Damasio, A. (1980) 'Anatomical Basis of Conduction Aphasia', *Brain*, *103*, 337–50
———, Damasio, A., Rizzo, M., Varney, N. and Gersh, F. (1982) 'Aphasia with Nonhemorrhagic Lesions in the Basal Ganglia and Internal Capsule', *Arch. Neurol*, *39*, 15–20
Darley, F., Aronson, A. and Brown, J. (1975) *Motor Speech Disorders*, Saunders, Philadelphia
David, A. and Bone, I. (1984) 'Mutism Following Left Hemisphere Infarction', *J. Neurol., Neurosurg., Psychiat.*, *47*, 1342–44
De Ajuriaguerra, J., Hécaen, H. and Angelergues, R. (1960a) 'Les Apraxies. Variétés Cliniques et Latéralisation Lésionelle', *Revue Neurol. (Paris)*, *102*, 566–94
———, Muller, M. and Tissot, R. (1960b) 'A Propos de quelques Problèmes Posés par

l'Apraxie dans les Démences', *Encéphale*, 5, 375–401
—— and Stambak, M. (1969) 'Developmental Dyspraxia and Psychomotor Disorders' in P. Vinken and G. Bruyn (eds), *Handbook of Clinical Neurology*, vol. 4, Elsevier, Amsterdam
—— and Stucki, J.-D. (1969) 'Developmental Disorders of the Body Schema', in P. Vinken and G. Bruyn (eds), *Handbook of Clinical Neurology*, vol. 4, Elsevier, Amsterdam
—— and Tissot, R. (1969) 'The Apraxias' in P. Vinken and G. Bruyn (eds), *Handbook of Clinical Neurology*, vol. 4, Elsevier, Amsterdam
Deal, J. and Darley, F. (1972) 'The Influence of Linguistic and Situational Variables on Phonemic Accuracy in Apraxia of Speech', *J. Speech Hear. Res.*, 15, 639–53
—— and Florance, C. (1978) 'Modification of the Eight Step Continuum for Treatment of Apraxia of Speech in Adults', *J. Speech Hear. Dis.*, 43, 1, 83–95
Denny-Brown, D. (1958) 'The Nature of Apraxia', *J. Nerv. Ment. Dis.*, 126, 9–33
Deodato, M., Di Rosa, A., Meduri, M. and Bramanti, P. (1979) 'Un Caso di Aprassia della Marcia: Considerazioni Clinico-Patogenetiche', *Acta Neurol. (Napoli)*, 39, 196–99
De Renzi, E. (1982) *Disorders of Space Exploration and Cognition*, Wiley, New York
—— (1985) 'Methods of Limb Apraxia Examination and their Bearing on the Interpretation of the Disorder' in E. Roy (ed.), *Neuropsychological Studies of Apraxia and Related Disorders*, Elsevier, Amsterdam
—— and Faglioni, P. (1967) 'The Relationship between Visuospatial Impairment and Constructional Apraxia', *Cortex*, 3, 327–42
——, Faglioni, P., Lodesani, M. and Vecchi, A. (1983) 'Impairment of Left Brain-damaged Patients on Imitation of Single Movements and Motor Sequences; Frontal and Parietal-injured Patients Compared', *Cortex*, 19, 333–43
——, Faglioni, P. and Sorgato, P. (1982) 'Modality-Specific and Supramodal Mechanisms of Apraxia', *Brain*, 105, 301–12
——, Motti, F. and Nichelli, P. (1980) 'Imitating Gestures: A Quantitative Approach to Ideomotor Apraxia', *Arch. Neurol.*, 37, 1, 6–10
——, Pieczuro, A. and Vignolo, L. (1966) 'Oral Apraxia and Aphasia', *Cortex*, 2, 50–73
——, Pieczuro, A. and Vignolo, L. (1968) 'Ideational Apraxia: A Quantitative Study', *Neuropsychologia*, 6, 41–52
Derouesne, J., Beauvois, M. and Ranty, C. (1977) 'Deux Composantes dans l'Articulation du Langage Oral: Preuve Experimentale de Leur Independence', *Neuropsychologia*, 15, 143–53
Deshayes, A., Cressard, P., Paulin, M., Berger, C. and Lebreton, C. (1979) 'Contribution à l'Étude de l'Apraxie Constructive dans les Lésions Hémisphériques Droites et Gauches' in P. Sizaret (ed.), *Comptes Rendus du Congrès de Psychiatrie et de Neurologie de Langue Française*, 77, vol. II, Masson, Paris
Deutsch, S. (1981) 'Oral Form Identification as a Measure of Cortical Sensory Dysfunction in Apraxia of Speech and Aphasia', *J. Comm. Dis.*, 14, 65–73
—— (1984a) 'Prediction of Site of Lesion from Speech Apraxic Error Patterns' in J. Rosenbek, M. McNeil and A. Aronson (eds), *Apraxia of Speech*, College-Hill, San Diego
—— (1984b) 'Oral Stereognosis' in C. Code *et al.* (eds), *Experimental Clinical Phonetics*, Croom Helm, Beckenham
Diller, L. and Gordon, W. (1981) 'Rehabilitation and Clinical Neuropsychology' in S. Filskov and T. Boll (eds), *Handbook of Clinical Neuropsychology*, Wiley, New York
Dowden, P., Marshall, R. and Tompkins, C. (1981) 'Amer-Ind Sign as a Communicative Facilitator for Aphasic and Apraxic Patients' in R. Brookshire (ed.), *Clinical Aphasiology, Conference Proceedings*, BRK, Minneapolis
Duensing, F. (1953) 'Raumagnostische und ideatorisch-apraktische Störung des gestaltenden Handelns', *Deutsche Zft. f. Nervenheilkunde*, 170, 72–94
Duffy, J. and Watkins, L. (1984) 'Effect of Response Choice Relatedness on Pantomime and Verbal Recognition Ability in Aphasic Patients', *Brain Lang.*, 21, 291–306

Dunlop, J. and Marquardt, T. (1977) 'Linguistic and Articulatory Aspects of Single Word Production in Apraxia of Speech', *Cortex, 13*, 1, 17–29

Edwards, M. (1984) *Disorders of Articulation*, Springer, Wien, New York

Estañol, B.V. (1981) 'Gait Apraxia in Communicating Hydrocephalus', *J. Neurol., Neurosurg. Psychiat., 44*, 305–08

Evarts, E. and Wise, S. (1984) 'Basal Ganglia Outputs and Motor Control' in CIBA *Foundation Symposium, 107*, 83–96

Faglioni, P. and Basso, A. (1985) 'Historical Perspectives on Neuroanatomical Correlates of Limb Apraxia' in E. Roy (ed.), *Neuropsychological Studies of Apraxia and Related Disorders*, Elsevier, Amsterdam

Ferrer-Abizanda, I., Alvarez, E.F., Gonzalez, A. and Pineda, M. (1977) 'Apraxia Oculomotora Congénita. A Propósito de Cuatro Observaciones', *Rev. Oto-Neuro-Oftalm., 35*, 43–48

Filskov, S. and Boll, T. (eds) (1981) *Handbook of Clinical Neuropsychology*, Wiley, New York

Fisher, M. (1956) 'Left Hemiplegia and Motor Impersistence', *J. Nervous and Mental Disease, 123*, 3, 201–18

Flechsig, P. (1901) 'Developmental (Myelogenetic) Localisation of the Cortex in Human Subjects', *Lancet*, Oct. 19, 1027–29

Florance, C., Rabidoux, P. and McCauslin, L. (1980) 'An Environmental Manipulation Approach to Treating Apraxia of Speech' in R. Brookshire (ed.), *Clinical Aphasiology, Conference Proceedings*, BRK, Minneapolis

Frederiks, J. (1985) 'Disorders of the Body Schema' in J. Frederiks (ed.), *Handbook of Clinical Neurology*, vol. 1 (45), Elsevier, Amsterdam

Freund, H-J. and Hummelsheim, H. (1984) 'Premotor Cortex in Man; Evidence for Innervation of Proximal Limb Muscles', *Exp. Brain Res, 53*, 479–82

Fromm, D., Abbs, J., McNeil, M. and Rosenbek, J. (1982) 'Simultaneous Perceptual-Physiological Method for Studying Apraxia of Speech', in R. Brookshire (ed.), *Clin. Aphasiology, Conf. Proceed.*, BRK, Minneapolis

Frostig, M. (1966) *Frostig Developmental Test of Visual Perception*, NFER, Windsor

Gainotti, G., Miceli, G. and Caltagirone, C. (1977) 'Constructional Apraxia in Left Brain-damaged Patients; A Planning Disorder?' *Cortex, 13*, 109–18

———— and Tiacci, C. (1970) 'Patterns of Drawing Disability in Right and Left Hemisphere Patients', *Neuropsychologia, 8*, 379–84

Gazzaniga, M. (1978) 'Is Seeing Believing? Notes on Clinical Recovery' in S. Finger (ed.), *Recovery from Brain Damage: Research and Theory*, Plenum, New York

————, Bogen, J. and Sperry, R. (1967) 'Dyspraxia Following Division of the Cerebral Commissures', *Arch. Neurol., 16*, June, 606–12

Gersh, F. and Damasio, A. (1981) 'Praxis and Writing of the Left Hand may be Served by Different Callosal Pathways', *Arch. Neurol., 38*, Oct., 634–36

Geschwind, N. (1965) 'Disconnexion Syndromes in Animals and Man', *Brain, 88*, 237–94, 585–644

Gittinger, J. and Sokol, S. (1982) 'Visual Evoked Potential in the Diagnosis of Congenital Ocular Motor Apraxia', *Amer. J. Ophthalmol, 93*, 6, 700–03

Godel, V., Nemet, P. and Lazar, M. (1979) 'Congenital Ocular Motor Apraxia', *Ophthalmologica, 179*, 2, 90–93

Golden, C. (1981) *Diagnosis and Rehabilitation in Clinical Neuropsychology*, Thomas, Springfield, Illinois

———— (1981a) A Standardized Version of Luria's Neuropsychological Tests: a Quantitative and Qualitative Approach to Neuropsychological Evaluation, in S. Filskov *et al.*, eds.

———— (1984) 'Controversial Therapies', *Pediatric Clinics of N. America, 31*, 2, 359–69

Goodglass, H. and Kaplan, E. (1983) *Assessment of Aphasia and Related Disorders*, 2nd edn, Lea & Febiger, Philadelphia

Goodnow, J. (1977) *Children's Drawing*, Fontana/Open Books, Glasgow
Gordon, N. and McKinlay, I. (eds) (1980) *Helping Clumsy Children*, Churchill, Edinburgh
Gresty, M., Halmagyi, G. and Taylor, D. (1983) 'Head Thrusting and Head Nodding in Children with Disturbances of Ocular Motility' in K. Wybar *et al.* (eds), *Paediatric Ophthalmology*, Marcel Dekker, New York
Grover, W., Tucker, S. and Wenger, D. (1978) 'Clinical Variations in two Children with Neuropathic Gaucher Disease', *Ann. Neurol.*, *3*, 281–83
Gubbay, S. (1975) *The Clumsy Child, A Study of Developmental Apraxia and Agnosic Ataxia*, Saunders, London
———— (1978) 'Management of Developmental Apraxia', *Devel. Med. Child Neurol.*, *20*, 643–46
Guyard, H., Sabouraud, O. and Gagnepain, J. (1981) 'A Procedure to Differentiate Phonological Disturbances in Broca's Aphasia and Wernicke's Aphasia', *Brain Lang.*, *13*, 19–30
Guyette, T. and Diedrich, W. (1981) 'Critical Review of Developmental Apraxia of Speech', *Speech and Language, Advances in Basic Research and Practice*, *5*, 1–49
Halpern, H., Darley, F. and Brown, J. (1973) 'Differential Language and Neurologic Characteristics in Cerebral Involvement', *J. of Speech and Hear. Dis.*, *38*, 162–73
———— Keith, R. and Darley, F. (1976) 'Phonemic Behaviour of Aphasic Subjects Without Dysarthria or Apraxia of Speech', *Cortex*, *12*, 365–72
Hartje, W., Kerschensteiner, M. und Sturm, W. (1975) 'Konstruktive Apraxie und räumliche Orientierungsstörung', *Aktuelle Neurologie*, *2*, 3, 179–87
Hartman, D. (1984) 'Neurogenic Dysphonia', *Ann Otol. Rhinol. Laryngol.*, *93*, 1, 57–64
Hécaen, H. and Albert, M. (1978) *Human Neuropsychology*, Wiley, New York
———— and Assal, G. (1970) 'Comparison of Constructive Deficits Following Right and Left Hemispheric Lesions', *Neuropsychologia*, *8*, 289–303
———— and De Ajuriaguerra, J. (1954) 'Balint Syndrome (Psychic Paralysis of Visual Fixation) and its Minor Forms', *Brain*, *77*, 373–400
————, Penfield, W., Bertrand, C. and Malmo, R. (1956) 'Syndrome of Apractognosia due to Lesions of the Minor Cerebral Hemisphere', *Arch. Neurol. Psychiat.*, *75*, 400–34
———— and Rondot, P. (1985) 'Apraxia as a Disorder of a System of Signs' in E.A. Roy (ed.), *Neuropsychological Studies of Apraxia and Related Disorders*, Elsevier, Amsterdam
Heilman, K. (1973) 'Ideational Dyspraxia — A Redefinition', *Brain*, *96*, 861–64
———— (1975) 'A Tapping Test in Apraxia', *Cortex*, *11*, 259–63
———— and Rothi, L. (1985) 'Apraxia' in K. Heilman and E. Valenstein (eds), *Clinical Neuropsychology*, 2nd edn, Oxford University Press, Oxford
————, Rothi, L. and Valenstein, E. (1982) 'Two Forms of Ideomotor Apraxia', *Neurology*, *32*, 4, 342–46
————, Schwartz, H. and Geschwind, N. (1975) 'Defective Motor Learning in Ideomotor Apraxia', *Neurology*, *25*, 1018–20
Henderson, S. and Hall, D. (1982) 'Concomitants of Clumsiness in Young Schoolchildren', *Devel. Med. Child Neurol.*, *24*, 448–60
Hijdra, A. and Meerwaldt, J. (1984) 'Balint's Syndrome in a Man with Border-zone Infarcts Caused by Atrial Fibrillation', *Clin. Neurol. Neurosurg.*, *86*, 1, 51–54
Hill, B. (1978) *Verbal Dyspraxia in Clinical Practice*, Pitman, Melbourne, Australia
Holle, B. (1976) *Motor Development in Children, Normal and Retarded*, Blackwell, Oxford
Holmes, G. (1938) 'Cerebral Integration of the Ocular Movements', *Brit. Med. J.*, *2*, 107–12
Hopkins, H. and Smith, H. (eds) (1983) *Occupational Therapy*, Lippincott, Philadelphia
Hrbek, A. (1977) 'Patofyzologická Interpretace a Klasifikace Apraxií', *Ceskoslovenská Neurologie a Neurochirurgie*, *40*, 1, 31–9
Hunt, R. and Cohen, D. (1984) 'Psychiatric Aspects of Learning Disabilities', *Pediatric Clinics of N. Amer.*, *31*, 2, 471–97
Hyvärinen, J. (1982) 'Posterior Parietal Lobe of the Primate Brain', *Physiological Reviews*,

62, 3, 1060–1129

Itoh, M. and Sasanuma, S. (1984) 'Articulatory Movements in Apraxia of Speech' in J. Rosenbek, M. McNeil and A. Aronson (eds), *Apraxia of Speech*, College-Hill, San Diego

———, Sasanuma, S., Hirose, H., Yoshioka, H. and Ushijima, T. (1980) 'Abnormal Articulatory Dynamics in a Patient with Apraxia of Speech: X-Ray Microbeam Observation', *Brain Lang.*, *11*, 66–75

———, Sasanuma, S. and Ushijima, T. (1979) 'Velar Movements During Speech in a Patient with Apraxia of Speech', *Brain Lang.*, *7*, 227–39

Jennett, B. and Teasdale, G. (1981) *Management of Head Injuries*, Davis, Philadelphia

Johnson, D. and Myklebust, H. (1967) *Learning Disabilities: Educational Principles and Practices*, Grune, New York

Johnston, C. and Diller, L. (1983) 'Error Evaluation Ability of Right-Hemisphere Brain-Lesioned Patients who have had Perceptual-Cognitive Retraining', *J. Clin. Neuropsychol.*, *5*, 4, 401–02

Jouandet, M. and Gazzaniga, M. (1979) 'The Frontal Lobes' in M. Gazzaniga (ed.), *Handbook of Behavioural Neurobiology, Volume 2: Neuropsychology*, Plenum, New York

Joynt, R., Benton, A. and Fogel, M. (1962) 'Behavioural and Pathological Correlates of Motor Impersistence', *Neurology (Minneap.)*, *12*, 876–81

Kaplan, E. (1977) 'Praxis: Development' in B. Wolman (ed.), *International Encyclopedia of Psychiatry, Psychology, Psychoanalysis and Neurology*, Von Nostrand, New York, pp. 26–29

Kaufmann, H. (1979) 'Zwillinge mit Kongenitaler Okulomotorischer Apraxie (Cogan-Syndrom)', *Klin. Mbl. Augenheilk*, *175*, 3, 360–66

Keatley, M. and Pike, P. (1976) 'An Automated Pulmonary Function Laboratory: Clinical Use in Determining Respiratory Variations in Apraxia' in R. Brookshire (ed.), *Clinical Aphasiology Conf. Proc.*, BRK, Minneapolis

Keiner, G. and Keiner, E. (1958) 'Congenital Ocular Motor Apraxia', *Am. J. Ophthal.*, *46*, 382–85

Keller, E. (1984) 'Simplification and Gesture Reduction in Phonological Disorders of Apraxia and Aphasia' in J. Rosenbek, M. McNeil and A. Aronson (eds), *Apraxia of Speech*, College-Hill, San Diego

Kelso, J. and Tuller, B. (1981) 'Toward a Theory of Apractic Syndromes', *Brain Lang.*, *12*, 2, 224–45

Kent, R. and Rosenbek, J. (1982) 'Prosodic Disturbance and Neurologic Lesion', *Brain Lang.*, *15*, 259–91

——— (1983) 'Acoustic Patterns of Apraxia of Speech', *J. Speech Hear. Res.*, *26*, 231–49

Kephart, N. (1971) *Slow Learner in the Classroom*, Merrill, Columbus, Ohio

Kerschensteiner, M. and Poeck, K. (1974) 'Bewegungsanalyse bei buccofacialer Apraxie', *Nervenarzt*, *45*, 9–15

———, Poeck, K. and Lehmkuhl, G. (1975) 'Die Apraxien', *Aktuelle Neurologie*, *2*, 3, 171–78

Kertesz, A. (1984) 'Subcortical Lesions and Verbal Apraxia' in J. Rosenbek, M. McNeil and A. Aronson (eds), *Apraxia of Speech*, College-Hill, San Diego

——— (1985) 'Apraxia and Aphasia: Anatomical and Clinical Relationship' in E.A. Roy (ed.), *Neuropsychological Studies of Apraxia and Related Disorders*, Elsevier, Amsterdam

——— and Ferro, J. (1984) 'Lesion Size and Location in Ideomotor Apraxia', *Brain*, *107*, 921–33

Kimura, D. (1977) 'Acquisition of a Motor Skill After Left-Hemisphere Damage', *Brain*, *100*, 527–42

——— (1982) 'Left-Hemisphere Control of Oral and Brachial Movements and their Relation to Communication', *Phil. Transacts. Royal Soc., London, B298*, 135–49

Klich, R., Ireland, J. and Weidner, W. (1979) 'Articulatory and Phonological Aspects of Consonant Substitutions in Apraxia of Speech', *Cortex*, *15*, 3, 451–70

Knuckey, N., Apsimon, T. and Gubbay, S. (1983) 'Computerised Axial Tomography in Clumsy Children with Developmental Apraxia and Agnosia', *Brain and Development*, 5, 1, 14–19

Knutsson, E. and Lying-Tunell, U. (1985) 'Gait Apraxia in Normal-pressure Hydrocephalus. Patterns of Movement and Muscle Activation', *Neurology*, 35, 155–60

Kohs, S. (1919) *Kohs Block Design Test*, NFER, Windsor

Kools, J. and Tweedie, D. (1975) 'Development of Praxis in Children', *Percept. Mot. Skills*, 40, 1, 11–19

Koppitz, E. (1964) *The Bender Gestalt Test for Young Children*, Grune, New York

Kretschmer, H. (1974) 'Callosal Tumours' in P. Vinken *et al.*, eds., *Handbook of Clinical Neurology*, Vol. 17

Lacks, P. (1984) *Bender Gestalt Screening for Brain Dysfunction*, Wiley, New York

Lakke, J., r.d. Burg, W. and Wiegman, J. (1982) 'Abnormalities in Postural Reflexes and Voluntarily Induced Automatic Movements in Parkinson Patients, *Clin. Neurol. Neurosurg.*, 84, 4, 227–35

———, van Weerden, T. and Staal-Schreinemachers, A. (1984) 'Axial Apraxia. A Distinct Phenomenon', *Clin. Neurol. Neurosurg.*, 86, 4, 291–94

La Pointe, L. and Wertz, R. (1974) 'Oral Movement Abilities and Articulatory Characteristics of Brain Injured Adults', *Perceptual and Motor Skills*, 39, 39–46

Larrabee, G., Levin, H., Huff, F., Kay, M. and Guinto, F. (1985) 'Visual Agnosia Contrasted with Visual-Verbal Disconnection', *Neuropsychologia*, 23, 1, 1–12

Laszlo, J. and Bairstow, P. (1985) *Perceptual-motor Behaviour: Developmental Assessment and Therapy*, Holt, Rinehart and Winston, New York

Lebrun, Y. (1982) 'Aphasie de Broca et Anarthrie', *Acta Neurol. Belg.*, 82, 80–90

Le Doux, J. (1979) 'Parietooccipital Symptomatology — The Split-Brain Perspective' in M. Gazzaniga (ed.), *Handbook of Behavioural Neurobiology, Volume 2, Neuropsychology*, Plenum, New York

Lefford, A., Birch, H. and Green, G. (1974) 'Perceptual and Cognitive Bases for Finger Localisation and Selective Finger Movement in Preschool Children', *Child Devel.*, 45, 335–43

Lehmkuhl, G. and Poeck, K. (1981) 'A Disturbance in the Conceptual Organisation of Actions in Patients with Ideational Apraxia', *Cortex*, 17, 1, 153–58

——— and Willmes, K. (1983) 'Ideomotor Apraxia and Aphasia: An Examination of Types and Manifestations of Apraxic Symptoms', *Neuropsychologia*, 21, 3, 199–212

Leischner, A. (1983) 'Side Differences in Writing to Dictation of Aphasics with Agraphia: A Graphic Disconnection Syndrome', *Brain Lang.*, 18, 1, 1–19

Lesný, I. (1978) 'Dětské Neobratnosti, Zvláštni Syndromy ve Skupině Lehkých Mozkových Dysfunkcí *Československá Psychiatrie*, 74, 3, 121–27

Levin, H. (1973) 'Motor Impersistence and Proprioceptive Feedback in Patients with Unilateral Cerebral Disease', *Neurology (Minneap.)*, 23, 833–41

Levine, D., Kaufman, K. and Mohr, K. (1978) 'Inaccurate Reaching Associated with a Superior Parietal Lobe Tumour', *Neurology*, 28, 556–61

Levine, M. and Zallen, B. (1984) 'The Learning Disorders of Adolescence: Organic and Nonorganic Failure to Strive', *Pediatric Clinics of N. America*, 31, 2, 345–69

Lezak, M. (1983) *Neuropsychological Assessment*, 2nd edn, Oxford University Press, Oxford

Lhermitte, F. (1983) '"Utilisation Behaviour" and its Relation to Lesions of the Frontal Lobes', *Brain*, 106, 237–55

Liepmann, H. (1908) *Drei Aufsätze aus dem Apraxiegebiet*, Karger, Berlin

Lubinski, R. (1981) 'Environmental Language Intervention' in R. Chapey (ed.), *Language Intervention Strategies in Adult Aphasia*, Wilkins, Baltimore/London

Luria, A. (1948, transl. 1963) *Restoration of Function after Brain Injury*, Pergamon, London

——— (1972) *The Man with a Shattered World*, Penguin, Harmondsworth

——— (1973) *The Working Brain*, Penguin, Harmondsworth

———— and Tsvetkova, L. (1964) 'The Programming of Constructive Activity in Local Brain Injuries', *Neuropsychologia, 1*, 1–14

———— and Yudovich, F. (1956, transl. 1971) *Speech and the Development of Mental Processes in the Child*, Penguin, Harmondsworth

Lyle, D. (1961) 'A Discussion of Oculomotor Apraxia with a Case Presentation', *Trans. Am. Ophthal. Soc., 59*, 274–85

MacKay, D. (1985) 'A Theory of Representation, Organisation and Timing of Actions, with Implications for Sequencing Disorders' in E.A. Roy (ed.), *Neuropsychological Studies of Apraxia and Related Disorders*, Elsevier, Amsterdam

Mackenzie, C. (1982) 'Aphasic Articulatory Defect and Aphasic Phonological Defect', *Brit. J. Disord. Communic., 17*, 1, 27–46

Mack, J. and Levine, R. (1981) 'The Basis of Visual Constructional Disability in Patients with Unilateral Cerebral Lesions', *Cortex, 17*, 4, 515–31

Margolin, D. (1984) 'Neuropsychology of Writing and Spelling: Semantic, Phonological, Motor and Perceptual Processes', *Qt. J. Exp. Psychol, 36A*, 3, 459–89

Marinkovic, S., Kovacevic, M. and Kostic, V. (1984) 'Isolated Occlusion of the Angular Gyri Artery — A Correlative Neurological and Anatomical Study — Case Report', *Stroke, 15*, 2, 366–70

Marquardt, T. and Sussman, H. (1984) 'The Elusive Lesion — Apraxia of Speech Link in Broca's Aphasia' in J. Rosenbek, M. McNeil and A. Aronson (eds), *Apraxia of Speech*, College-Hill, San Diego

Marsden, C. (1984) 'Which Motor Disorder in Parkinson's Disease Indicates the True Motor Function of the Basal Ganglia?' in *CIBA Foundation Symposium, 107*, 225–37

Martin, A. (1974) 'Objections to the Term Apraxia of Speech', *J. Speech Hear. Disorders, 39*, 1, 53–64

———— and Rigrodsky, S. (1974) 'An Investigation of Phonological Impairment in Aphasia', Part 1, *Cortex, 10*, 317–28

Mateer, C. (1978) 'Impairments of Non-verbal Oral Movements after Left-hemisphere Damage: A Follow-up Analysis of Errors', *Brain Lang., 6*, 334–41

———— and Kimura, D. (1977) 'Impairment of Non-verbal Oral Movements in Aphasia', *Brain Lang., 4*, 262–76

McLean, P. (1972) 'Cerebral Evolution and Emotional Processes: New Findings on the Striatal Complex', *Ann. N.Y. Acad. Sciences, 193*, 137–49

Megna, G., Bandiera, L., Nardulli, R., Del Prete, M., Basalisco, G. and Coratelli, A. (1979) 'Osservazioni sull' Atassia Ottica con Turbe Aprassiche e dell'Orientamento Spaziale Attraverso lo Studio Longitudinale di Due Casi', *Acta Neurol. (Napoli), 39*, 191–95

Messerli, P. (1983) 'De l'Aphemie à l'Apraxia of Speech, où les Tribulations d'une Notion' in P. Messerli, P. Lavorel and J.-L. Nespoulous (eds), *Neuropsychologie de l'Expression Orale*, Editions du Centre National de la Recherche Scientifique, Paris

Meyer, J. and Barron, D. (1960) 'Apraxia of Gait: A Clinico-Physiological Study', *Brain, 83*, 261–83

Meyer-Probst, B., Heider, B., Cammann, G. and Engel, H. (1980) 'Erfahrungen mit dem Dysraxie-Test (nach Lesný)', *Psychiat. Neurol. Med. Psychol. (Leipzig), 32*, 1, 46–53

Miller, E. (1984) *Recovery and Management of Neuropsychological Impairments*, Wiley, New York

Mills, R. and Swanson, P. (1978) 'Vertical Oculomotor Apraxia and Memory Loss', *Annals of Neurology, 4*, 2, 149–53

Mitchell, J. (1976) 'Three-Dimensional Construction Tests for Children Five to Six Years', *Am. J. Occupational Therapy, 30*, 6, 362–9

Mohr, J. (1980) 'Revision of Broca Aphasia and the Syndrome of Broca's Area Infarction and its Implications in Aphasia Theory' in R. Brookshire (ed.), *Clinical Aphasiology, Conference Proceedings*, BRK, Minneapolis

————, Pessin, M., Finkelstein, S., Funkelstein, H., Duncan, G. and Davis, K. (1978)

'Broca Aphasia: Pathologic and Clinical', *Neurology (Minneap.)*, 28, 311-24
Monaco, F., Pirisi, A., Sechi, G. and Cossu, C. (1980) 'Acquired Ocular-Motor Apraxia and Right-sided Cortical Angioma', *Cortex*, 16, 1, 159-67
Monrad-Krohn, G. (1947) 'Dysprosody or Altered Melody of Language', *Brain*, 70, 405-15
Moore, W., Rosenbek, J. and La Pointe, L. (1976) 'Assessment of Oral Apraxia in Brain Injured Adults' in R. Brookshire (ed.), *Clinical Aphasiology: Conference Proceedings*, BRK, Minneapolis
Morlaas, J. (1928) *Contribution à l'Étude de l'Apraxie*, Legrand, Paris
Naeser, M., Alexander, M., Helm-Estabrooks, N., Levine, H., Laughlin, S. and Geschwind, N. (1982) 'Aphasia with Predominantly Subcortical Lesion Sites', *Arch. Neurol.*, 39, 2-14
Nakatani, T., Watanabe, J., Tashiro, T., Takeishi, S., Takeishi, G., Hosoda, K. and Uemura, K. (1984) 'Case of Post-traumatic Interhemispheric Disconnection Syndrome (Japanese)', *No To Shinkei*, 36, 1, 65-71
Narbona, J., Crisci, C. and Villa, I. (1980) 'Familial Congenital Ocular Motor Apraxia and Immune Deficiency' (letter to ed.), *Arch. Neurol.*, 37, 325
Neetens, A. and Rubbens, M. (1982) 'Congenital Ocular Motor Apraxia', *Bull. Soc. belge, Ophthal.*, 203, 71-74
Nespoulous, J.-L., Lecours, A. and Joanette, Y. (1983) 'La Dichotomie 'Phonetique-Phonemique', a-t-elle une Valeur Neurologique' in P. Messerli, P. Lavorel and J.-L. Nespoulous (eds), *Neuropsychologie de l'Expression Orale*, Editions du Centre National de la Recherche Scientifique, Paris
Newcombe, F. and Ratcliff, G. (1979) 'Long-term Psychological Consequences of Cerebral Lesions' in M. Gazzaniga (ed.), *Handbook of Behavioural Neurobiology, Vol. 2, Neuropsychology*, Plenum Press, New York
Newhoff, M., Florance, C., Malone, P., Ritter, G. and Webster, E. (1980) 'Home and Family; Problems and Payoffs. A Panel Presentation and Discussion' in R. Brookshire (ed.), *Clinical Aphasiology, Conference Proceedings*, BRK, Minneapolis
Ohigashi, Y., Hamanaka, T., Ohashi, H., Hadano, K., Kato, N., Tomita, A. and Asano, K. (1980) 'A Propos de l'Hétérogénéité de l'Apraxie Bucco-faciale', *Folia Psychiat. et Neurol. Japonica*, 34, 1, 35-43
O'Malley, P. and Griffith, J. (1977) 'Perceptuomotor Dysfunction in the Child with Hemiplegia', *Devel. Med. Child, Neurol.*, 19, 172-78
Orrison, W. and Robertson, W. (1979) 'Congenital Ocular Motor Apraxia: A Possible Disconnection Syndrome', *Arch Neurol.*, 36, 1, 29-31
Osterrieth, P. (1944) 'Le Test de Copie d'une Figure Complexe', *Archs. de Psychol.*, 30, 206-356
Overton, W. and Jackson, J. (1973) 'Representation of Imagined Objects in Action Sequences: A Developmental Study', *Child Devel.*, 44, 309-14
Perenin, M.T. and Vighetto, A. (1983) 'Optic Ataxia: A Specific Disorder in Visuomotor Co-ordination' in A. Hein and M. Jeannerod (eds), *Spatially Oriented Behaviour*, Springer, New York
Piaget, J. (1936, transl. 1977) *Origin of Intelligence in the Child*, Penguin, Harmondsworth
―――― and Inhelder, B. (1956) *The Child's Conception of Space*, Routledge, London
Pieczuro, A. and Vignolo, L. (1967) 'Studio Sperimentale sull'Aprassia Ideomotoria', *Sistema Nervoso*, 19, 131-43
Piercy, M., Hécaen, H. and De Ajuriaguerra, J. (1960) 'Constructional Apraxia Associated with Unilateral Cerebral Lesions, Left and Right Sided Cases Compared', *Brain*, 83, 225-42
―――― and Smyth, V. (1962) 'Right Hemisphere Dominance for certain Non-Verbal Intellectual Skills', *Brain*, 85, 775-90
Poeck, K. (1975) 'Neuropsychologische Symptome ohne eigenständige Bedeutung', *Aktuelle Neurologie*, 2, 3, 199-208
―――― (1982) 'Two Types of Motor Apraxia', *Arch. Ital. Biol.*, 120, 1/3, 361-69

———— (1983) 'Ideational Apraxia', *J. Neurol, 230*, 1, 1–5
———— and Kerschensteiner, M. (1971) 'Ideomotor Apraxia Following Right-sided Cerebral Lesion in a Left-handed Subject', *Neuropsychologia, 9*, 359–61
———— and Lehmkuhl, G. (1980a) 'Das Syndrom der ideatorischen Apraxie und seine Lokalisation', *Nervenarzt, 51*, 217–25
———— and Lehmkuhl, G. (1980b) 'Ideatory Apraxia in a Left-handed Patient with Right-sided Brain Lesion', *Cortex, 16*, 2, 273–84
————, Lehmkuhl, G. and Willmes, K. (1982) 'Axial Movements in Ideomotor Apraxia', *J. Neurol. Neurosurg. Psychiat., 45*, 1125–29
———— and Orgass, B. (1964) 'Die Entwicklung des Körperschemas bei Kindern im Alter von 4-10 Jahren', *Neuropsychologia, 2*, 109–30
———— and Orgass, B. (1966) 'Gerstmann's Syndrome and Aphasia', *Cortex, 2*, 421–37
———— and Orgass, B. (1971) 'The Concept of the Body Schema: A Critical Review and Some Experimental Results', *Cortex, 7*, 254–77
Rabidoux, P., Florance, C. and McCauslin, L. (1980) 'The Use of a Handi Voice in the Treatment of a Severely Apractic, Non-Verbal Patient' in R. Brookshire (ed.), *Clinical Aphasiology, Conference Proceedings*, BRK, Minneapolis
Reason, J. (1979) 'Actions not as Planned' in G. Underwood *et al.* (eds), *Aspects of Consciousness*, Academic Press, London
Rendle-Short, J., Appleton, B. and Pearn, J. (1973) 'Congenital Ocular Motor Apraxia. Paediatric Aspects', *Austral. Paediat. J., 9*, 263–68
Roberts, J. (1984) *Differential Diagnosis in Neuro-psychiatry*, Wiley, New York
Robles, J. (1966) 'Congenital Ocular Motor Apraxia in Identical Twins', *Arch. Ophthal, 75*, 746–49
Roeltgen, D. (1985) 'Agraphia' in K. Heilman and E. Valenstein (eds), *Clinical Neuropsychology*, 2nd edn, Oxford University Press, Oxford
———— and Heilman, K. (1983) 'Apractic Agraphia in a Patient with Normal Praxis', *Brain Lang., 18*, 35–46
————, Sevush, S. and Heilman, K. (1983) 'Pure Gerstmann's Syndrome from a Focal Lesion', *Arch. Neurol., 40*, Jan., 46–47
Rosenbek, J., Kent, R. and La Pointe, L. (1984) 'Apraxia of Speech: An Overview and Some Perspectives' in J. Rosenbek, M. McNeil and A. Aronson (eds), *Apraxia of Speech*, College-Hill, San Diego
————, Lemme, M., Ahern, M., Harris, E. and Wertz, R. (1973) 'A Treatment for Apraxia of Speech in Adults', *J. Speech Hear. Dis., 38*, 4, 462–72
————, McNeil, M., Teetson, M., Odell, K. and Collins, H. (1981) 'A Syndrome of Neuromotor Speech Deficit and Dysgraphia?' in R. Brookshire (ed.), *Clinical Aphasiology, Conference Proceedings*, BRK, Minneapolis
Rosenthal, M., Griffith, E., Bond, M. and Miller, J. (1983) *Rehabilitation of the Head-Injured Adult*, Davis, Philadelphia
Rothi, L. and Heilman, K. (1985) 'Ideomotor Apraxia: Gestural Discrimination, Comprehension and Memory' in E.A. Roy (ed.), *Neuropsychological Studies of Apraxia and Related Disorders*, Elsevier, Amsterdam
———— and Horner, J. (1983) 'Restitution and Substitution: Two Theories of Recovery with Application to Neurobehavioural Treatment', *J. Clin. Neuropsychol., 5*, 1, 73–81
Roy, E.A. (1978) 'Apraxia: A New Look at an Old Syndrome', *J. Human Movement Studies, 4*, 191–210
———— (1981) 'Action Sequencing and Lateralised Cerebral Damage: Evidence for Asymmetrics in Control' in J. Long *et al.* (eds), *Attention and Performance*, Lawrence Erlbaum, Hillsdale
———— (1982) 'Action and Performance' in A. Ellis (ed.), *Normality and Pathology in Cognitive Functions*, Academic Press, London
———— (1983) 'Neuropsychological Perspectives on Apraxia and Related Action Disorders' in R. Magill (ed.), *Memory and Control of Action*, North Holland, Amsterdam, pp.

293-320
—— and Square, P. (1985) 'Common Considerations in the Study of Limb, Verbal and Oral Apraxia' in E.A. Roy (ed.), *Neuropsychological Studies of Apraxia and Related Disorders*, Elsevier, Amsterdam
Samson, M., Mihout, B., Proust, B. and Parain, D. (1983) 'Apraxie Oculomotrice Congénitale, Deux Cas avec Étude Électro-oculographique', *Rev. Neurol. (Paris), 139*, 515-18
Sands, E., Freeman, P. and Harris, K. (1978) 'Progressive Changes in Articulatory Patterns in Verbal Apraxia: A Longitudinal Case Study', *Brain Lang., 6*, 97-105
Sandyk, R. (1983) 'Parkinsonism, Gait Apraxia and Dementia Associated with Intracranial Calcifications', *S. Afric. Med., J., 63*, 7, 738-39
Seinsch, W. (1981) 'Artikulatorische Dyspraxie. Eine Störung des Bewegungsentwurfs im Broca-Assoziationscortex', *Folia Phoniat, 33*, 125-30
Semenza, G., Denses, G., D'Urso, V., Romano, O. and Montorsi, T. (1978) 'Analytic and Global Strategies in Copying Designs by Unilaterally Brain-damaged Patients', *Cortex, 14*, 401-10
Shankweiler, D. and Harris, K. (1966) 'An Experimental Approach to the Problem of Articulation in Aphasia', *Cortex, 2*, 277-87
—— and Taylor, M. (1968) 'Electromyographic Studies of Articulation in Aphasia', *Arch. Phys. Med. Rehab., 49*, 1-8
Sheridan, M. (1975) *Children's Developmental Progress*, NFER, Windsor
Siev, E. and Freishtat, B. (1976) *Perceptual Dysfunction in the Adult Stroke Patient*, Charles B. Slack Inc., USA
Signoret, J.-L. and North, P. (1979) 'Les Apraxies Gestuelles' in P. Sizaret (ed.), *Comptes Rendus du Congrès de Psychiatrie et de Neurologie de Langue Française, 77*, vol. II, Masson, Paris
Small, L. (1982) *The Minimal Brain Dysfunctions: Diagnosis and Treatment*, Free Press, New York/London
Smith, M. (1979) 'The Edinburgh Stroke Rehabilitation Study', *Brit. J. Occup. Therapy, 42*, 6, 139-42
Spreen, O. and Gaddes, W. (1967) *Developmental Norms for Fifteen Neuropsychological Tests, Age Six to Fifteen*, University of Victoria, Australia, Neuropsychology Laboratory
Square, P, Darley, F. and Sommers, R. (1981) 'Speech Perception Among Patients Demonstrating Apraxia of Speech, Aphasia and Both Disorders' in R. Brookshire (ed.), *Clinical Aphasiology Conference Proceedings*, BRK, Minneapolis
—— (1982) 'Analysis of the Productive Errors made by Pure Apractic Speakers with Differing Loci of Lesions' in R. Brookshire (ed.), *Clinical Aphasiology Conference Proceedings*, BRK, Minneapolis
—— and Mlcoch, A. (1983) 'Syndrome of Subcortical Apraxia of Speech: An Acoustic Analysis (Abstract)' in R. Brookshire (ed.), *Clinical Aphasiology Conference Proceedings*, BRK, Minneapolis
Stanton, K., Yorkston, K., Kenyon, V. and Beukelman, D. (1981) 'Language Utilization in Teaching Reading to Left Neglect Patients' in R. Brookshire (ed.), *Clinical Aphasiology, Conference Proceedings*, BRK, Minneapolis
Stern, Y., Mayeux, R., Rosen, J., Ilsen, J. (1983) 'Perceptual Motor Dysfunction in Parkinson's Disease', *J. Neurol. Neurosurg. Psychiat., 46*, 145-51
Sugishita, M., Toyokura, Y., Yoshioka, M. and Yamada, R. (1980) 'Unilateral Agraphia after Section of the Posterior Half of the Truncus of the Corpus Callosum', *Brain Lang., 9*, 215-25
Tansley, A. (1980a) *Motor Education*, Arnold, Leeds
—— (1980b) *Perceptual Training*, Arnold, Leeds
Taylor, D. (1980) 'Disorders of Head and Eye Movements in Children', *Trans. Ophthal. Soc. UK., 100*, 489-94
Taylor, R. and Warren, S.A. (1984) 'Educational and Psychological Assessment of Children

with Learning Disorders', *Pediatric Clinics of N. Amer., 31*, 2, 281–96

Thomsen, I.V. (1984) 'Late Outcome of Severe Blunt Head Trauma: a 10-15 Year Follow-Up', *J. Neurol. Neurosurg. Psychiat., 47*, 3, 260–68

Thursfield, D. (1980) 'Psychiatry' in N. Gordon and I. McKinlay (eds), *Helping Clumsy Children*, Churchill, Edinburgh

Tognola, G. and Vignolo, L. (1980) 'Brain Lesions Associated with Oral Apraxia in Stroke Patients: A Clinico-neuro-radiological Investigation with the CT Scan', *Neuropsychologia, 18*, 257–72

Tonkovich, J. and Marquardt, T. (1977) 'Effects of Stress and Melodic Intonation on Apraxia of Speech' in R. Brookshire (ed.), *Clinical Aphasiology Conference Proceedings*, BRK, Minneapolis

Touwen, B. and Prechtl, H. (1970) *The Neurological Examination of the Child with Minor Nervous Dysfunction*, Heinemann, London

Trevarthen, C. (1984) 'How Control of Movement Develops' in H. Whiting (ed.), *Human Motor Actions: Bernstein Reassessed*, Elsevier, North Holland

Trost, J. and Canter, G. (1974) 'Apraxia of Speech in Patients with Broca's Aphasia, A Study of Phoneme Production Accuracy and Error Patterns', *Brain Lang., 1*, 63–79

Truelle, J.-L., Fardoun, R., Delestre, F., Cottenceau, C.-N., Maubert, M., Rieux, D., Travers, M,-A. and Derouesne, C. (1979) 'L'Apraxie d'Origine Frontale' in P. Sizaret (ed.), *Comptes Rendus du Congrès de Psychiatrie et de Neurologie de Langue Française, 77*, vol. II, Masson, Paris

Tyler, H.R. (1969) 'Defective Stimulus Exploration in Aphasic Patients', *Neurology, 19*, 2, 105–12

Vassella, F., Lütschg, J. and Mumenthaler, M. (1972) 'Cogan's Congenital Ocular Motor Apraxia in two Successive Generations', *Devel. Med. Child Neurol., 14*, 788–803

Villardita, C., Smirni, P., Le Pira, F., Zappala, G. and Nicoletti, F. (1982) 'Mental Deterioration, Visuoperceptive Disabilities and Constructional Apraxia in Parkinson's Disease', *Acta Neurol. Scandinav., 66*, 112–20

Volpe, B., Sidtis, J., Holtzman, J., Wilson, D. and Gazzaniga, M. (1982) 'Cortical Mechanisms Involved in Praxis: Observations Following Partial and Complete Section of the Corpus Callosum in Man', *Neurology, NY, 32*, 654–50

Vygotsky, L. (1934, transl. 1962), *Thought and Language*, MIT, Cambridge, Massachusetts

Walton, J., Ellis, E. and Court, S. (1962) 'Clumsy Children: Developmental Apraxia and Agnosia', *Brain, 85*, 603–12

Warren, M. (1981) 'Relationship of Constructional Apraxia and Body Scheme Disorders to Dressing Performance in Adult CVA', *Am. J. Occup. Ther., 35*, 7, 431–37

Warrington, E. (1969) 'Constructional Apraxia' in P. Vinken and G. Bruyn (eds), *Handbook of Clinical Neurology, Volume 4*, Elsevier, Amsterdam

——, James, M. and Kinsbourne, M. (1966) 'Drawing Disability in Relation to Laterality of Lesion', *Brain, 89*, 53–82

—— and James, M. (1967) 'Disorders of Visual Perception in Patients with Localised Cerebral Lesions', *Neuropsychologia, 5*, 253–66

Watamori, T., Itoh, M., Fukusako, Y. and Sasanuma, S. (1981) 'Oral Apraxia and Aphasia', *Ann. Bull. Res. Inst. Logopedics and Phoniatrics, 15*, 129–46

Watson, R. and Heilman, K. (1983) 'Callosal Apraxia', *Brain, 106*, 391–403

Weinberg, J., Diller, L., Gordon, W., Gerstman, L., Lieberman, A., Lakin, P., Hodges, G. and Ezrachi, O. (1977) 'Visual Scanning Training Effect on Reading-Related Tasks in Acquired Right Brain Damage', *Arch. Phys. Med. Rehabil., 58*, 479–86

—— (1979) 'Training Sensory Awareness and Spatial Organisation in People with Right Brain Damage', *Arch. Phys. Med. Rehabil., 60*, 491–96

Wertz, R. (1984) 'Response to Treatment in Patients with Apraxia of Speech' in J. Rosenbek, M. McNeil and A. Aronson (eds), *Apraxia of Speech*, College-Hill, San Diego

——, La Pointe, L. and Rosenbek, J. (1984) *Apraxia of Speech in Adults. The Disorder and its Management*, Grune, New York

Whitaker, H. (1983) 'Towards a Brain Model of Automatisation: A Short Essay' in R. Magill (ed.), *Memory and Control of Action*, North Holland, Amsterdam

Williams, N. (1967) 'Correlation Between Copying Ability and Dressing Activities in Hemiplegia', *Am. J. Phys. Med.*, *46*, 4, 1332–40

Worrall, E. and Gillham, R. (1983) 'Lithium-induced Constructional Dyspraxia', *Brit. Med. J.*, *286*, January, p. 189

Yakovlev, P. and Lecours, A. (1967) 'The Myelogenetic Cycles of Regional Maturation of the Brain' in A. Minkowski (ed.), *Regional Development of the Brain in Early Life*, Blackwell, Oxford

Yarbus, A. (1967) *Eye Movements and Vision*, Plenum, New York

Young, G., Collins, D. and Hren, M. (1983) 'Effect of Pairing Scanning Training with Block Design Training in the Remediation of Perceptual Problems in Left Hemiplegics', *J. Clin. Neuropsychol. 5*, 3, 201–12

Zaidel, D. and Sperry, R. (1977) 'Some Long-term Motor Effects of Cerebral Commissurotomy in Man', *Neuropsychologia, 15*, 193–204

Zangwill, O. (1960) 'Le Problème de l'Apraxie Idéatoire', *Rev. Neurol. (Paris), 102*, 595–603

Zaret, C., Behrens, M. and Eggers, H. (1980) 'Congenital Ocular Motor Apraxia and Brainstem Tumour', *Arch. Ophthalmol.*, *98*, 2, 328–30

Zee, D., Yee, R. and Singer, H. (1977) 'Congenital Ocular Motor Apraxia', *Brain, 100*, 3, 581–99

AUTHOR INDEX

Abbs, J. 97
Abercrombie, M. 157
Adams, R. 125–6
Agostoni, E. 39, 88
Ahern, M. 110
Akelaitis, A. 132
Albert, M. 8, 28, 80–1, 83, 106, 136, 140, 214
Alexander, M. 45–6, 104
Alvarez, E. 119
Angelergues, R. 1
Appleton, B. 117
Apsimon, T. 160
Araie, M. 117
Aram, D. 156, 166, 167
Archer, L. 111
Arena, R. 63, 76
Arnheim, D. 155, 165, 183, 186–7
Aronson, A. 90
Arrigoni, G. 62, 64
Arthuis, M. 123
Asano, K. 229
Assal, G. 36, 66, 70, 74
Auerbach, S. 45–6
Awaya, Y. 117
Ayres, A. 119, 121, 155–6, 162, 164, 166, 183, 186–7, 211

Badian, N. 176
Bairstow, P. 183
Baker, J. 187
Baloh, O. 123
Bandiera, L. 46
Barbizet, J. 128–33
Barranger, J. 123
Barron, D. 143, 145–8
Basalisco, G. 228
Basso, A. 10, 37, 39
Baum, B. 152
Beauvois, M. 107
Behrens, M. 122
Benson, D. 1, 45, 81, 83, 87, 214
Benton, A. 43, 60–1, 63, 84, 178
Ben-Yishay, Y. 43–4
Berger, C. 223
Bergès, J. 167

Bernard, B. 63–4
Bertrand, C. 56
Beukelman, D. 205
Birch, H. 167
Black, F. 63–4, 87–8
Blum, C. 78, 142
Blumstein, S. 96
Boder, E. 123
Bogen, J. 128, 131, 134–5
Boll, T. 10, 13
Boller, F. 88
Bollier, B. 110
Bond, M. 195, 213
Bone, I. 92
Borden, G. 102
Botez, M. 46
Bower, T. 172–3
Bowman, C. 52
Bradley, L. 174
Bramanti, P. 223
Brion, S. 132–3
Brown, J. 7, 10, 18, 24–5, 28–9, 39, 41, 49, 52, 54, 56, 78, 88, 90, 105, 131, 142, 154, 160–1, 182, 214
Bruininks, R. 165
Buckingham, H. 91, 96, 107–8
Burr, L. 170, 186–7

Cahn, L. 187
Caltagirone, G. 67
Cambier, J. 43, 88
Cammann, G. 166
Canter, G. 95–6
Carecchi, A. 119, 125
Carr, J. 195
Cermak, S. 155–6, 164–6, 168, 179, 182
Chartier, B. 220
Christensen, A-L. 13–14
Chu, F. 121, 123
Cicci, R. 174
Cogan, D. 115–16, 120–3, 125–6
Cohen, D. 189
Coletti, A. 39
Collins, D. 212

235

Conrad, K. 166–9, 179
Consoli, S. 60, 62, 66, 77
Coratelli, A. 228
Cossu, C. 125
Cottenceau, C-N. 232
Court, S. 155
Cressard, P. 75
Crisci, C. 123
Cummings, J. 87

Dabul, B. 100
Damasio, A.H. 45, 104, 107, 131, 136
Darley, F. 90, 92, 95–6, 100–2, 105
David, A. 92
Davis, K. 229
De Ajuriaguerra, J. 1, 7, 13, 22, 24–5, 28, 37, 39, 40, 46, 63, 77–8, 87–8, 127, 150, 152, 156, 159, 169, 178, 183
Deal, J. 95, 110
Decroix, J. 43
Degos, J-D. 220
Delestre, F. 88, 136
Del Prete, M. 228
Denes, G. 77
Denny-Brown, D. 24, 41, 125, 141–2, 146, 148
Deodato, M. 145–6
De Renzi, E. 1, 7, 11, 13, 22–8, 30, 37, 39–40, 46, 51–3, 56, 58, 62–4, 66, 76, 125, 127, 166, 197
Derouesne, J. 107
Deshayes, A. 75
Deutsch, S. 98, 107, 211
Diedrich, W. 156, 167, 179
Diller, L. 43, 195, 197, 203
Di Rosa, A. 145
Dowden, R. 111
Drake, C. 166, 168
Duensing, F. 66, 69, 70, 77
Duffy, J. 11, 13, 203
Duizabo, P. 128
Duncan, G. 229
Dunlop, J. 95
D'Urso, V. 77

Edwards, M. 102
Eggers, H. 122
Elghozi, D. 43
Ellis, E. 155
Engel, H. 228
Estañol, B. 154–6

Evarts, E. 148
Ezrachi, O. 232

Faglioni, P. 10, 23, 27–8, 37, 58, 62–4
Fardoun, R. 88, 136
Ferrer, I. 119–20, 123
Ferro, J. 37
Filskov, S. 10
Finkelstein, S. 90
Fisher, M. 43
Flechsig, P. 160
Florance, C. 109–11
Fogel, M. 43, 60–1, 63, 178
Frederiks, J. 152
Freeman, F. 95
Freishtat, B. 212
Freund, H-J. 141
Fromm, D. 97
Frostig, M. 170
Fukusako, Y. 77
Funkelstein, H. 229

Gaddes, W. 178
Gagnepain, J. 100, 107
Gainotti, G. 63, 66–7, 69, 71, 74, 76, 119, 125
Gazzaniga, M. 128–9, 136, 140, 206
Gersh, F. 131
Gerstman, L. 43
Geschwind, N. 7, 10, 27, 37, 54, 141–2, 148
Gillham, R. 88
Gittinger, J. 118
Godel, V. 121–3
Golden, C. 13, 187, 195
Gonzalez, A. 224
Goodglass, H. 11, 29, 30, 59, 101, 103, 106, 137
Goodnow, J. 172
Gordon, N. 155, 164, 166, 183, 186–7, 190–1
Gordon, W. 195, 197
Graveleau, P. 43
Green, G. 167
Gresty, M. 122
Griffith, E. 195
Griffith, J. 157
Grover, W. 123
Gubbay, S. 155, 157, 160, 164, 166, 170, 190
Guinto, F. 227
Guyard, H. 100, 107

Guyette, T. 156, 167, 179

Hass, A. 221
Hadano, K. 229
Hall, D. 164, 166, 178
Hall, K. 152
Halmagyi. G. 122
Halpern, H. 96, 105
Hamanaka, T. 27
Harris, E. 230
Harris, K. 95, 97
Hartje, W. 66, 152
Hartman, D. 92, 105
Hécaen, H. 1, 8, 28, 46, 56, 63, 66, 70, 74, 80, 106, 127, 136, 140, 214
Heider, B. 166
Heilman, K. 7, 10-13, 24, 27-9, 36-7, 80-1, 83-4, 128-9, 131, 134-5, 141, 197, 199, 203, 211
Helm-Estabrooks, N. 104
Henderson, S. 164, 166, 178
Hijdra, A. 127
Hill, B. 110, 112
Hirose, H. 98
Hodges, G. 232
Hodges, J. 187
Hodson, B. 52
Holle, B. 171-2
Holmes, G. 127
Holtzman, J. 128
Hopkins, H. 195
Horner, J. 197
Hrbek, J. 10
Hren, M. 212
Huff, F. 36
Hummelsheim, H. 141
Hunt, R. 189
Hyvärinen, J. 56, 87, 127

Ilson, J. 231
Inhelder, B. 172
Ireland, J. 96
Itoh, M. 27, 98

Jackson, J. 168
James, M. 58, 76
Jedynak, C-P. 132-3
Jennett, B. 195, 213
Joanette, Y. 107
Johnson, D. 183, 186-7
Johnston, C. 203
Jouandet, M. 136, 140
Joynt, R. 43

Kaplan, E. 11, 29, 30, 59, 101, 103, 106, 137, 168, 169, 179
Kato, N. 229
Kaufman, K. 45
Kaufmann, H. 117, 121
Kay, M. 227
Keatley, M. 98
Keefe, N. 88
Keiner, G. 118, 121-2
Keith, R. 96
Keller, E. 95, 108
Kelso, J. 91, 102
Kent, R. 91, 97, 105
Kenyon, V. 205
Kephart, N. 119, 121, 186-7
Kerschensteiner, M. 30, 34, 39, 40, 48-9, 51-3, 66, 147, 197
Kertesz, A. 13, 37, 98
Kimura, D. 7, 13, 27-8, 39, 52-4, 100, 102, 108, 198-9
Kinsbourne, M. 58
Klich, R. 96
Knuckey, N. 160, 190
Knutsson, E. 143, 145-6, 149
Kohs, S. 60, 170
Kools, J. 166
Koppitz, E. 174
Kostic, V. 87
Kovacevic, M. 87
Kretschmer, H. 128, 135

Lacks, P. 58, 62, 174
Lakin, P. 232
Lakke, J. 141, 2
La Pointe, L. 47, 52, 91
Larrabee, G. 36, 79
Laszlo, J. 183
Laughlin, S. 229
Lazar, M. 121
Leader, B. 77, 142
Lebreton, C. 223
Lebrun, Y. 90
Lecours, A. 107, 160
Le Doux, J. 78
Lefford, A. 167
Lehmkuhl, G. 13, 18, 20-5, 27, 29, 30, 34-5, 39, 40, 141, 198
Leischner, A. 78
Lejeune, A. 128
Lemme, M. 110
Le Pira, F. 88
Lesný, I. 166
Levin, H. 36, 43

Levine, D. 45
Levine, M. 188
Levine, R. 60, 62–3, 69, 77
Lesak, M. 10, 61, 174
Lézine, I. 167
Lhermitte, F. 43, 137
Lieberman, A. 232
Liepmann, H. 9, 10, 18, 37, 40, 54
Lodesani, M. 28
Lubinski, R. 109
Luria, A. 1, 7, 13, 14, 16, 46, 88,
    90, 94, 107, 126, 136, 140, 148,
    160–2, 205, 207–8, 216
Lütschg, J. 118
Luzzatti, C. 37
Lying-Tunnell, U. 143, 145–6, 148
Lyle, D. 122–3

McKay, D. 20
Mack, J. 60, 62–3, 69, 77
Mackenzie, C. 107
Malone, P. 109
Margolin, D. 83, 174
Marinkovic, S. 87
Marquardt, T. 95, 98, 111
Marsden, C. 149
Marshall, R. 111
Martin, A. 96
Masson, M. 222
Mateer, C. 52–3, 100, 102, 108
Maubert, M. 232
Mayeux, R. 148
McCauslin, L. 109, 111
McKinlay, I. 155, 164, 166, 183,
    186–7, 190–1
McLean, P. 160
McNeil, M. 96–7, 104
Meduri, M. 145
Meerwaldt, J. 127
Megna, G. 46
Messerli, P. 90
Meyer, J. 143, 145–8
Meyer-Probst, E. 166, 168
Miceli, G. 67
Mihout, B. 116
Miller, E. 195, 197
Miller, J. 195
Mills, R. 125
Mitchell, J. 176, 178
Mlcoch, A. 94, 98
Mohr, J. 45, 90, 98, 112
Monaco, F. 125–6
Monrad-Krohn, G. 94

Montorsi, T. 231
Moore, W. 47
Morlaas, J. 23
Motti, P. 1, 13, 28, 30
Muller, M. 24
Mumenthaler, M. 118
Mykelbust, H. 183, 186–7

Nauser, M. 104
Nakatani, T. 128
Narbona, J. 123
Nardulli, R. 46
Nation, J. 156, 166–7
Neetens, A. 123
Nemet, P. 121
Nespoulous, J-L. 107
Newcombe, F. 10, 61
Newhoff, M. 109
Nichelli, F. 232
North, P. 6, 11, 17, 23, 25, 27–9, 56,
    78

Ohashi, H. 27
Ohigashi, Y. 27, 53, 108
O'Malley, P. 157
Orgass, B. 84, 152–3, 168
Orlando, G. 39
Orrison, W. 117–18, 120–3
Osterrieth, P. 58
Overton, W. 168
Ozawa, T. 117

Parain, D. 116
Passafiume, D. 88
Paulin, M. 75
Pearn, J. 117
Penfield, W. 56
Perenin, M. 46
Pessin, M. 90
Piaget, J. 142, 158–9, 172
Pieczuro, A. 1, 13, 22, 26–7, 29, 30,
    51
Piercy, M. 63, 67, 76
Pike, P. 98
Pineda, M. 224
Pirisi, A. 125–6
Poeck, K. 13, 18, 20–5, 27, 30, 34,
    39, 40, 48–9, 51–3, 84, 141–2,
    148, 152–3, 168, 197–8
Prechtl, H. 178
Proust, B. 116

Rabidoux, P. 109, 111

Ranty, C. 107
Ratcliff, G. 11, 61
Reason, J. 20
Regli, F. 36-7
Reingold, D. 121, 123
Rendle-Short, J. 117, 123
Rieux, D. 232
Rigrodsky, S. 96
Ritter, G. 229
Rizzo, M. 104
Roberts, J. 11
Robertson, W. 117-18, 120-3
Robles, J. 121, 123
Roeltgen, D. 83-4, 141, 214
Rogers, K. 221
Romano, O. 231
Rondot, P. 8, 28
Rosen, J. 148
Rosenbek, J. 47, 91, 96-7, 104-5, 110
Rosenthal, M. 10, 195, 197
Rothi, L. 7, 10-12, 27-8, 36, 80, 197, 199
Roy, E. 7, 20, 25, 27-8, 36, 39, 54, 91, 96, 108, 136, 148, 197-9, 203, 211
Rubbens, M. 123

Sabouraud, O. 100, 107
Samson, M. 116, 118-20, 122-3
Sands, E. 95
Sandyk, R. 145-6
Sasanuma, S. 98
Schwartz, H. 27
Sechi, G. 125-6
Seinsch, W. 92
Semenza, C. 77
Sevush, S. 84
Shankweiler, D. 95, 97
Shepherd, R. 195
Sheridan, M. 171-2
Sidtis, J. 128
Siev, E. 212
Signoret, J-L. 6, 11, 17, 23, 25, 27-9, 56, 78
Simpson, R. 52
Sinclair, W. 155, 165, 183, 186-7
Singer, H. 116
Small, L. 164, 183, 185, 189-90
Smirni, P. 88
Smith, H. 195
Smith, M. 10, 202
Smyth, V. 76

Sokol, S. 118
Sommers, R. 92, 102
Sorgato, P. 23, 27, 37
Sperry, R. 128, 130
Spinnler, H. 37
Spreen, O. 178
Square, P. 7, 39, 54, 91-2, 94, 96, 98, 102, 107
Staal-Schreinemachers, A. 141
Stambak, M. 156, 159, 178, 183
Stanton, K. 205
Stern, Y. 148
Strub, R. 63, 87-8
Strube, E. 43
Stucki, J-D. 152, 169
Sturm, W. 66
Sugishita, M. 131
Sussman, H. 98
Swanson, P. 125

Takeishi, S.G. 229
Tansley, A. 187
Tashiro, T. 128
Taylor, D. 97
Taylor, R. 170
Teasdale, G. 195, 213
Teetson, M. 104
Thomsen, I. 213
Thursfield, D. 189
Tiacci, C. 66, 69, 71, 76
Tissot, R. 7, 24, 28, 78
Tognola, G. 13, 54
Tomita, A. 229
Tompkins, C. 111
Tonkovich, J. 111
Touwen, B. 178
Toyokura, Y. 131
Travers, M-A. 232
Tredici, G. 220
Trevarthen, C. 158, 173
Trost, J. 95-6
Truelle, J-L. 88, 136
Tsai, S. 87
Tsvetkova, L. 88
Tucker, S. 123
Tuller, B. 91, 102
Tweedie, D. 166
Tyler, H. 84, 119, 126

Uemura, K. 229
Ushijima, T. 98

Valenstein, E. 7, 28
v.d. Burg, W. 141

v. Weerden, T. 141
Vassella, F. 118, 121–3
Vecchi, A. 28
Vighetto, A. 46
Vignolo, L. 1, 13, 22, 26–7, 29, 30, 51, 54
Villa, I. 123
Villardita, C. 88
Volpe, B. 128, 134
Vygotsky, L. 161–2

Walton, J. 155
Warren, M. 152–3
Warren, S. 170
Warrington, E. 56, 58, 66, 69, 70, 76–7
Watamori, T. 27, 47–9, 53, 108
Watanabe, J. 128
Watkins, L. 11, 13, 203
Watson, R. 128–9, 131–2, 134–5
Webster, E. 229
Weidner, W. 96
Weinberg, J. 207, 212
Wenger, D. 123

Wertz, R. 47, 52, 100–1, 105, 108–9, 111–13
Whitaker, H. 91, 94, 142
Wiegman, J. 141
Williams, N. 152
Willmes, K. 13, 27, 141
Worrall, E. 88
Wise, S. 148

Yakovlev, P. 160
Yarbus, A. 84, 119, 126
Yee, R. 16, 123
Yorkston, K. 205
Yoshioka, M.H. 131
Young, G. 212
Yudovich, F. 126, 161

Zaidel, D. 130
Zallen, B. 188
Zangwill, O. 24
Zappala, G. 232
Zaret, C. 122–3
Zasetsky, L. 1, 16, 46, 216
Zee, D. 116–17, 119

SUBJECT INDEX

agnosia 217
    finger 84, 133, 152, 167–8
    object use, 21, 23–4
    simultanagnosia 80, 126
    visual 79–80, 127
agraphia *see* dysgraphia
akinetic mutism 92, 135, 140
alexia *see* dyslexia
alien hand 132
Alzheimers disease *see* dementia
amnesic dyspraxia 52, 128
angular gyrus syndrome 87
aphasia *see* dysphasia
apractagnosia 3, 56, 136, 130, 164,
    183
apraxia *see* dyspraxia
apraxia of speech
    assessment 99–103
    associated disorders 104–8
    auditory perception 102
    clinical description 92–4, 99
    definition 90, 99
    developmental 156, 167
    differential diagnosis 92, 101–2,
        104–8
    dysarthria and 98, 102, 104–5, 112
    dysphasia and 96, 98, 103, 105–8
    error description 95–7
    instrumental description 97–8
    intonation in 93–4, 97, 110–11
    lesions in 98, 107–8
    linguistuc description 95–7, 103
    oral dyspraxia and 51, 94, 112
    oral stereognosis 102
    prognosis 102–3, 111–13
    theoretical issues 90–1, 96
    therapy 103, 108–13, 209
assessment 2–3, 8–13, 21–2, 27–9,
    47, 196–8
    see also differential diagnosis *and*
        the individual dyspraxias
associated disorders 14–15
    see also agnosia, dysphasia, space
        and the individual dyspraxias
ataxia 4, 119–20, 123, 135, 145–7
    see also frontal ataxia

axial dyspraxia
    assessment 141
    clinical descriptions 140–1
    definitions 141
    theoretical issues 141–2
    whole body movements 141, 144
    see also gait dyspraxia *and*
        parkinsonism

body awareness 36, 118–19, 152–4,
    159, 167, 169, 185
    see also space

callosal dyspraxia
    alien hand 132
    associated disorders 132, 135
    bimanual co-ordination 131–3
    constructional dyspraxia 78, 129,
        131
    dyscopia 131
    dysgraphia 130–1
    ideomotor dyspraxia 130
    lesions in 128, 134
    prognosis 129–31, 134–5
    proximal versus distal 130–1
    see also dysphasic dyspraxia,
        diagnostic dyspraxia *and*
        unilateral dyspraxia
classification of the dyspraxias 6–10,
    16, 128
clinical presentation 2–3, 212–13
    see also the individual dyspraxias
Cogan's syndrome 115
constructional dyspraxia
    assessment: left v. right hemisphere
        60, 67–70; qualitative 65–70;
        quantitative 63–5; three
        dimensional 60; two
        dimensional 58
    associated disorders 77, 79–85,
        126, 135, 150–3
    callosal dyspraxia and 78, 131
    clinical description 56–8, 85–7
    definition 56, 169
    dementia and 84
    developmental 169

differential diagnosis 57, 79–85
dressing and 151–3
dyscopia 131
error description 62; left v. right
    hemisphere 66–70; validity of
    70–6
ideational dyspraxia and 77–8
ideomotor dyspraxia and 77
incidence 77–8
lesions in 87–8, 131
theoretical issues 63, 76–9
therapy 79, 197, 205, 211
unilateral 129, 131
visual perception and 169
see also angular gyrus syndrome,
    Gerstmann's syndrome, space
counterholding 42, 145, 148

defining dyspraxias 1–8, 14–16,
    141–2, 147–9, 151–7, 212
see also individual dyspraxias
dementia and the dyspraxias 6, 14,
    22–4, 84, 109, 212
developmental dyspraxia
    anatomical-physiological
        considerations 157–61
    assessment 162–7, 176–9, 186
    associated disorders 156–7, 176
    constructional 167, 169–74, 176–8
    defining 155–7, 182
    descriptions of 155–7, 182, 190–4
    differential diagnosis 162–5,
        177–9, 182, 186
    dysgraphia and 171–6
    error description 167–8
    gestural 167–9
    graphic skills 171, 173–6
    hand-eye co-ordination 173–4
    incidence 190
    intelligence in 157, 166
    lesions in 123–4, 157, 160, 190
    perception and 156, 159
    prognosis 190
    theoretical issues 155, 157, 167,
        184–5, 194
    therapy 161–3, 179–83; counselling
        180, 188–9; programming 183–7
    see also ocular motor dyspraxia,
        praxis, space
diagnostic dyspraxia 132
differential diagnosis 2–6, 14–15,
    212–13
    see also assessment *and the*

    individual dyspraxias
disconnection hypothesis 9–10, 36–7,
    128–9
disconnection syndrome *see* callosal
    dyspraxia
dressing dyspraxia
    associated disorders 150
    body image and 152–4
    clinical description 137, 149–50
    constructional dyspraxia and 151–3
    incidence 150
    lesions in 150
    non-unitary disorder 151
    theoretical issues 151–3
    therapy 205–6, 208–9
dyscalculia 84, 134, 150, 176
dysgraphia 42, 217
    apraxia of speech and 94
    callosal lesions and 130–1
    developmental 171
    dyslexia and 83
    dysphasic 83, 175
    dyspraxic 82–3, 131, 174–6
    frontal 137
    hemiplegic writing 142, 214
    spatial 81, 126, 135, 150, 175
    therapy 205, 207, 214–15
dyslexia 81, 118–19, 126, 134, 150,
    217
dysphasia 217
    dyspraxia and 11–13, 94, 141
    optic 37
    visual scanning and 119, 126
    see also apraxia of speech,
        language, oral dyspraxia
dysphasic dyspraxia 130–1
dyspraxia
    apraxia versus 3–4
    praxia versus 4, 8
    *see separate headings and/or
        individual dyspraxias for:*
        assessment; associated
        disorders; classification; clinical
        presentation; definitions of;
        dementia and; differential
        diagnosis; dysphasia and; error
        types; incidence; intelligence
        and; language and; learning
        and; lesions in; manual
        dexterity and; motor
        development and; movement
        disorders and; psychiatric
        disorder and; theoretical issues;

underlying problems

echopraxia 126, 138
error recognition 18, 21, 28–9, 66,
    137, 140
  therapy and 112, 203
error types 6, 61, 168
  see also differential diagnosis,
    underlying disorder *and*
    individual dyspraxias
error utilisation 140, 203
eupraxis 4
eye control *see* ocular motor dyspraxia

facial dyspraxia *see* oral dyspraxia
finger agnosia 84, 133, 152, 167–8
foreign accent syndrome 94
frontal ataxia 146–7
frontal gait disturbance 126, 146, 148
  see also gait dyspraxia
frontal lobe syndrome 88, 136, 140,
    150
frontal dyspraxia
  assessment 14, 136, 138
  associated disorders 136, 138
  clinical description 136–40
  error description 136–40
  theoretical issues 136, 140
  therapy 198, 205

gait dyspraxia
  assessment 143
  associated disorders 135, 144–7
  axial movements in 144
  clinical description 143–6
  definitions 146–8
  differential diagnosis 146
  parkinsonism and 148–9
  theoretical issues 147–9
  see also axial dyspraxia
gaze dyspraxia *see* ocular motor
    dyspraxia
Gegenhalten 42, 145, 148
Gerstmann's syndrome 84
grasp reflex 41, 135, 144
groping reflex 41, 135

ideational dyspraxia
  assessment 20–2, 24
  associated disorders 22, 126
  clinical descriptions 17, 19
  constructional dyspraxia and 77–8
  definitions 9, 17, 23–5

dementia and 22, 24
differential diagnosis 17–18, 22,
    28, 42
  error description 17–20
  ideomotor dyspraxia and 17–18,
    25, 27–8
  incidence 22
  lesions in 22–3
  perception in 21, 203
  theoretical issues 21, 23–5
  therapy 198, 205–6
ideomotor dyspraxia
  assessment 26–7, 29–30, 141
  associated disorders 40, 77, 126
  clinical description 26
  definition 25–6
  differential diagnosis 28, 33, 36,
    40–6, 153
  error description 30–6
  ideational dyspraxia and 17–18, 25,
    27–8
  incidence 37–40
  learning in 27, 36
  lesions in 37–40
  perception and 28–9
  therapy 28, 35, 198–9
  unilateral 37, 130
  see also callosal, oral *and*
    sympathetic dyspraxia
incidence 1
  see also individual dyspraxias
innervatory dyspraxia 40
intelligence and dyspraxia 14, 157,
    166

language and dyspraxia 13, 51–4, 103,
    105–8, 126, 161
  see also dysphasia
learning and dyspraxia 27–8, 36
left–right orientation *see* space
lesions in dyspraxia 4
  see also subcortex *and* individual
    dyspraxias
limb kinetic dyspraxia 9, 40–1, 105
localisation *see* lesions

magnetic dyspraxia 42, 125, 141, 146
manual dexterity and dyspraxia 13–14,
    41–2, 150, 158, 179, 182
melokinetic dyspraxia 40
modality specific dyspraxias 27, 36–7,
    130
motor development 118, 158, 165

motor dyspraxia 40
motor impersistence 43, 135
movement disorders and dyspraxia 4,
   141–2, 147–9

neglect 81, 135, 140, 153
   see also space

ocular motor dyspraxia
   acquired 125–7, 135, 144
   congenital: assessment 115–19;
      associated disorders 119–20;
      clincial description 115–19;
      definition 115; differential
      diagnosis 122–4; error
      description 115–17; intelligence
      and 119–20; lesions in 123–4;
      motor development and 118;
      perception 119; prognosis
      121–4; reading 118–21;
      theoretical issues 117, 120,
      124; therapy 121
optic aphasia 36–7, 79
optic apraxia 37
optic ataxia 44–6, 127
   see also reaching
oral dyspraxia
   apraxia of speech and 51, 94,
      101–2, 112
   assessment 44, 47, 102
   associated disorders 40–4
   clinical description 47–51
   definition 46–7
   dysphasia and 51–4
   error description 47–51, 53–4
   lesions in 54–5, 108
   theoretical issues 51, 101–2, 108
   therapy 101–2, 110
orofacial dyspraxia *see* oral dyspraxia

parapraxia 7, 30, 34, 41, 49, 218
parkinsonism 88, 104, 141, 148–9
perception 5, 119, 156–9, 169, 172
   therapy and 211–12
   see also apractagnosia, space *and*
      individual dyspraxias
planning dyspraxia 126, 136, 156,
   161, 164
   see also frontal dyspraxia
praxis 8
   development of 118–19, 156–61,
      169
   language and 13, 140, 161

see also motor development
prognosis *see* therapy *and individual*
   dyspraxias
psychiatric disorders and dyspraxia 6,
   57, 93, 132, 140, 213
   see also dementia

reaching 44–6, 118–20, 124, 126,
   145, 173
reading *see* dyslexia
recovery *see* prognosis
reflexes and dyspraxia
   abnormal 41–3, 142, 148
   normal 3, 5, 117, 126, 158
remediation *see* therapy *and* individual
   dyspraxias
repellent dyspraxia 42, 125, 141, 146
right–left orientation *see* space

sensory perception *see* perception
space
   Euclidean 7, 78, 217
   extrapersonal 28, 56, 119, 152–9,
      167–9, 185
   intrapersonal 7, 28, 56, 119,
      152–6, 159
   neglect 80–1, 84, 135, 140, 150–3
   perception of 150
   pseudoneglect 133
   right–left orientation 84, 150,
      152–3, 167
   topographical 81, 127, 218
   see also agnosia, body awareness,
      dressing dyspraxia *and*
      perception
split brain *see* callosal dyspraxia
subcortex and dyspraxia 39, 88, 98,
   142, 148–9, 156
sympathetic dyspraxia 9, 27, 37

theoretical issues 6–9, 16, 128, 142,
   147–8
   see also individual dyspraxias
therapy
   ADL 10, 61, 199, 210
   aids 199, 210
   aims 196, 215, 216
   colour coding 208–9
   computers 210–11
   content of 61, 184, 216
   context of 195–6
   counselling 188–9, 212–13
   cure versus care 196–7

environmental structuring 209
error recognition 28–9, 35, 203–4
error utilisation 203–4
grading 198
guided imagery 209
issues in 184–5
landmarks 206–8
perceptual 185, 211–12
prognosis 204
programming 199–203
recovery 195–7
relearning in 36, 134, 199
skills versus processes 184–5
targeting behaviours 198
task construction 196, 199–203
techniques 199
theoretical issues 195–8, 211, 216
transfers 199
underlying problems 197–8
verbal support 134, 204–6

visual support 134, 206–9
writing 205, 207, 214–15
see also individual dyspraxias

underlying problems
acquired 7–10, 13, 76–9, 128–9,
140–2, 148–51
developmental 117, 156, 164, 169,
181–2
therapy and 197–8, 209
see also individual dyspraxias
unilateral dyspraxia 9, 27, 37, 41,
129–31
utilisation behaviour 43, 137

verbal dyspraxia *see* apraxia of speech
visual–spatial perception *see* perception

walking *see* gait dyspraxia
writing *see* dyspraxia, therapy